Building a High-Value Health System

BUILDING A HIGH-VALUE HEALTH SYSTEM

Rifat Atun and Gordon Moore

OXFORD
UNIVERSITY PRESS

Oxford University Press is a department of the University of Oxford. It furthers the University's objective of excellence in research, scholarship, and education by publishing worldwide. Oxford is a registered trade mark of Oxford University Press in the UK and certain other countries.

Published in the United States of America by Oxford University Press
198 Madison Avenue, New York, NY 10016, United States of America.

Library of Congress Cataloging-in-Publication Data
Names: Atun, Rifat, editor. | Moore, Gordon, editor.
Title: Building a high-value health system / [edited by] Professor Rifat Atun and Professor Gordon Moore.
Description: New York, NY : Oxford University Press, [2021] | Includes bibliographical references and index.
Identifiers: LCCN 2020049688 (print) | LCCN 2020049689 (ebook) | ISBN 9780197528549 (paperback) | ISBN 9780197528563 (epub) | ISBN 9780197528570 (online)
Subjects: MESH: Delivery of Health Care—methods | Systems Analysis | Health Planning—methods | Organizational Innovation
Classification: LCC RA418 (print) | LCC RA418 (ebook) | NLM W 84.1 | DDC 362.1—dc23
LC record available at https://lccn.loc.gov/2020049688
LC ebook record available at https://lccn.loc.gov/2020049689

DOI: 10.1093/med/9780197528549.001.0001

9 8 7 6 5 4 3 2 1

Printed by Marquis, Canada

CONTENTS

PREFACE

A growing challenge to all population-based health systems—whether nations or large organizations—is how to make healthcare delivery effective, efficient, equitable, satisfying, and, especially, affordable. The size of the task is clear. In the past 50 years, healthcare expenditures in the countries of the Organization for Economic Cooperation and Development countries have doubled to reach an average of around 10% of the gross domestic product (GDP) while that in the United States has trebled to reach above 18% of GDP, in excess of $3.5 trillion each year. Through 2040, projected per capita expenditure on healthcare in developed countries is estimated to exceed the rate of GDP growth. Who bears this increasing cost, and how, varies considerably among countries.

Delivery of healthcare services differs widely across the world. Benefits, results, and popular acceptance are markedly different. Countries have different mixes of public health services, high-quality medical care, level of personal financial risk protection and affordability, and national satisfaction. Most countries and businesses are struggling to find an equilibrium between benefits that are optimal for them and their constituents and the best value-for-money. No country would claim to have successfully achieved the perfect balance.

All health systems are in flux. Science is advancing our understandings of biology and, with it, the need will increase for health system reform to ensure their optimal use. New treatments, diagnostics, health technologies, and medicines will become available, contributing to rising medical care costs. Confronted by these costs, every population-based health system will seek to be more effective and efficient, while maintaining its acceptability to the population it serves. Inevitably, however, nations and organizations will be forced to face the fact that costs of health care will continue to increase and ultimately become unsustainable; countries will need to choose between other health and societal priorities and the extent and scope of medical care provided to citizens. Our hope in this workbook is to help decision makers learn to do this well.

Our goal in *Building a High-Value Population Health System* is to teach how a population can get better health for the amount it spends. The learning objectives are to prepare readers to understand a health system, create a strategic plan to improve it, and design actions to build a better system that improves care for populations. The educational process will provide tools and help readers to acquire skills and knowledge. Throughout, we treat population health as complex systems and show that using systems theory approaches can stimulate deep learning and transformative innovation.

Our population targets for health system improvement are middle- and high-income nations with adequate organizational and economic capacity to build a full-service health system. Despite the magnitude of the health system design challenge, there is no how-to book that describes and teaches a practical, general approach to designing anew or improving upon a current health system. We hope this workbook can meet that need.

This educational workbook focuses primarily on national systems of health care for populations and individuals. We recognize that public health and social determinants of health also have profound effects on the health of populations and must be considered part of achieving a high quality, equitable, and affordable health system. Public health can rightly claim equal or greater causality in global trends in health and disease in the past 100 years than the contribution of medical care. Social determinants such as economic success have been major factors in improving health. How much improvement each has contributed to the current state of health in developed countries has not been computed convincingly. For sure, public health and social determinants are important. But because individual healthcare services are high cost and have grown fastest, they have been more prominent in politics and government policy. Since medical care has directly consumed much more of countries' national resources, it is our primary concern in this workbook about policy development, change, and implementation.

The book's targeted audience is health system learners at all levels. Primary among them are teachers and students at medical, allied health professions, and public health school levels. Educators can use this workbook to teach their students how any health system works and how to improve it. It is designed to be used in classroom settings as the basis for a general course on teaching how to understand and improve healthcare. To make the book easy-to-use for educational purposes, we have highlighted educational instructions for students and teachers throughout. These sections are featured in italics.

This book will be of interest to other audiences as well, including business managers, delivery system leaders, politicians and their staff, and policymakers. Because the book is structured to catalyze strategic action, it will assist organizational change agents in designing and implementing plans to improve the cost, quality, and outcomes of their health system. For all readers, we hope that the book will be useful as a primer to enable them to plan and deliver a health system that works for them.

Using an active, learner-directed teaching method, the workbook systematically leads the reader through the steps of designing a system to fit a population's needs. The book lays out a general approach to analyzing a country's or organization's health system performance, evaluating the needs of the population to be served, assessing the key capacities available, and determining how to develop and implement health system design options that fit and are feasible. Students engage in a real planning process. The book will use case examples from across the globe to illustrate how all health systems are constructed, operate, and succeed or fail.

In Chapter 1, we present a definition of a health system. Following this, a distinction is drawn between a descriptive view of a *system* as a set of elements comprising the inputs, structure, and processes that deliver health outputs to a defined population and a *systems* analytical approach by which we examine, interpret, and seek to understand the complex interdependent, interactive, dynamic complexity of the system-in-action to produce the outcomes predetermined by its deep structure.

We introduce our framework for analyzing a health system in Chapter 2. The framework enables students to dissect the context, functions, outputs, and outcomes of a national health system. The students select a country that they will work on for the remainder of the course. They join a small group that shares the target country. In individual and small group work, they start a descriptive analysis of the health system of their selected country. Their work culminates in a presentation of the structure, goals, and results of each selected country to the entire group of students.

In Chapter 3, the students are presented with a historical perspective of health system development. We describe four major trends in healthcare globally over past 60 years to understand how we got to where we are today and to identify some of the challenges that await us.

In Chapter 4, the students formulate a vision and high-level goals for their country. In the process, they examine gaps between desired and actual outcomes in their country. By identifying strengths and weaknesses, opportunities and threats and by putting their country through an analysis of 12 parameters of performance, the students create a map demonstrating the largest performance gaps, which in turn leads them to identify the values, goals, and tentative objectives of their chosen country.

The students identify areas for change in Chapter 5. Returning to a systems thinking approach, each student identifies, describes, and justifies a policy, structure, or process change whose projected output is an improvement toward a desired health system goal. The students present and critique their ideas and identify one proposal to be carried forward collectively by their small group.

Chapter 6 guides each student through a number of tests to assess their plan's rationale, feasibility, and likely impact. The students present their ideas for group critique and collectively finalize one proposal that their group will take forward for implementation.

Chapter 7 reviews major learning insights generated in the workbook by the use of a systems thinking approach to analysis and planning. The systems archetype called 'The Tragedy of the Commons' is described, and value-for-money is redefined and enriched. Examples are given of health system interventions that represent three change models: single- and double-loop learning and fundamental reconceptualization.

Chapter 8 asks each student group to develop a proposed implementation plan. They examine their proposed change for its rationale, likely outcomes, and risks and consider how to achieve strategic change to ensure implementation happens. This process culminates in a presentation to the entire group, in which each small group argues for funding for their idea. Students will act as individual policymakers and select the proposals in which they would invest.

Chapter 9 concludes the book with a summary of the major challenges to all health systems in middle- and high-income countries and an integration of the interventional themes available to improve them. It ends with a summary of some suggestions of reconceptualized health systems and the skills, tools, and roles of design leaders in improving health systems to ensure their sustainability in the future.

ACKNOWLEDGMENTS

We would like to thank our publisher, Oxford University Press, and our editors, Sarah Humphreville and Emma Hodgdon, for helping us move our manuscript through to publication. In addition, we greatly appreciate the support of Harvard University's T. H. Chan School of Public Health, Harvard Medical School, and the Harvard Pilgrim Healthcare Institute. We are grateful for our many students, whose study with us over the years has stimulated the underlying educational methods in this workbook and improved our teaching. Thank you to our colleagues who have encouraged, participated, and critiqued our work, leading to and improving many of the ideas and methods in this workbook. We are grateful for the many researchers, healthcare organizations, and thought leaders who have shared insights with us and told their stories. We especially want to thank England's NHS and New England's Harvard Pilgrim Health Care, Atrius Health, and Harvard Vanguard Medical Associates for enabling each author to directly experience the satisfaction and tribulations of delivering primary care services to real people. Finally, we give special thanks to Mary Ellis, a recent honors graduate of the College of Arts and Sciences at Washington University in St. Louis, whose diligent review, critical comments, and valuable insights have made this a better book.

CHAPTER 1

Introduction to the Health of a Population

If I had one hour to save the world, I would spend fifty-five minutes defining the problem and only five minutes finding the solution.

—Albert Einstein

The purpose of this chapter is to help the reader understand the physiology of health systems as dynamic systems. We describe two ways we will view a health system.

First, we discuss health systems: how health systems are defined, depicted, and analyzed. We use the term *system* in this book to describe an interconnected set of component parts that form a dynamic whole. Each element has particular properties and characteristics, as does the whole. We present a high-level framework for understanding the component parts of a nation's health system.

Second, we introduce the idea of looking at health systems through the approach of *systems thinking*. In particular, in this chapter we present health systems as complex dynamic systems. In this view, a health system is examined as a complex set of interacting and interdependent processes.

THE HEALTH OF A NATION

What Determines Health?

The overall health of a population is the result of the interaction of many variables, of which healthcare services is but one. Health and well-being are influenced by many other factors—culture, education, income levels, gender, social behaviors, the environment, and economics, to name but a few. The model in Figure 1.1 categorizes these multiple drivers of health.

Modern societies have developed many interventions to improve the health and function of their constituents. Among the most visible influences on health are health services. These range from those provided to the entire population to those targeting individuals and families. Foremost among these are public health services and medical care. We also refer to the latter as medical services, individual healthcare services, or personal healthcare services. These two types of services—public health and medical care—have developed over time, energized by the specific intent to improve the health of the population.

At the population level, health systems have provided public health programs and services. These services target individual and collective health, usually through functions complementary to medical care. Public health programs are whole-population interventions that address health-related factors such as the environment (e.g., water and shelter), nutrition (healthy eating), and social factors (like violence and substance abuse), in

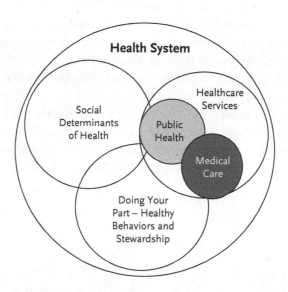

Figure 1.1 Determinants of health.

addition to providing general prevention strategies (such as vaccination and health education). Public health programs have had major impacts through managing epidemics, curbing substance abuse and smoking, promoting automobile safety, and educating the public about physical abuse and gun violence. In addition, public health has made the environment safer through clean water, adequate food and shelter, and safety in workplaces. In complementing medical care, public health has promoted prevention and early detection, vaccination, health education, and public policy changes (such as laws about smoking cessation or seatbelts) to encourage individuals to practice healthy behaviors and to protect their health.

Public health is the most cost-effective of health interventions. It is our view that public health has not only contributed mightily to the levels of health in all countries but that it also represents the most value-added way to improve health in the future for all nations. We see whole-population threats as the most significant future risks to health in middle- and high-income countries. Most important among these are lifestyle-related damage, violence and armed conflict, poverty, and climate change. The latter is, in our view, the most important future threat to the health of all nations through its direct effects influencing the physical environment, and causing severe weather events like flooding, drought, and fires. The consequent impact on natural ecosystems reduces food production and stimulates mass migration as well as triggering epidemics through the widening range of transmittable disease vectors.

Medical care is delivered to individuals and directed to their specific needs. Medical services consist of interventions that provide detection, diagnosis, and treatment of individual disease as well as those that aim to enhance wellness and well-being and prevent the development of illness. Middle- and high-income countries have all sought to provide some level of personal medical care.

In virtually all health systems, medical care is based on the Western model called "allopathic medicine." This model is science-based and is often referred to as "modern medicine," to contrast with homeopathy, folk, or traditional medicine. Allopathic medicine utilizes doctors, nurses, and other healthcare professionals to deliver modern surgery, medical diagnosis, treatment, and care in a variety of delivery modalities, ranging from primary care offices to telemedicine to technically sophisticated hospitals.

Individual healthcare services have not been limited to medical care. Multiple independent entities deliver individual healthcare services ranging from support services to Alcoholics Anonymous for alcoholics and other addictions, and lay support groups for mental health. However, our primary focus is on the formal structures of the medical care in middle- and high-income countries, comprising doctors, nurses, other healthcare professionals, hospitals, primary healthcare, insurers, payers, and those organized interventions that are designed to care for individuals.

Three categories of factors outside healthcare delivery also have significant effects on health. First, social determinants of health, such as education, housing, income, food access, employment, and work conditions, are broad societal factors that affect health status. Second, as shown in our model, we point out the important category of each individual's responsibility for their own and the collective health of the nation. Individual responsibility is significantly influenced by social determinants of health, as personal agency over one's health can vary with societal values, political milieu, socioeconomic status, racial background, geographic location, and other factors. However, individuals do bear some personal responsibility for their lifestyle behaviors, as well as for the appropriate use and stewardship of the medical and public health systems in which they participate. Third, environmental factors in the built environment or worsening natural habitats for humans, animals, and plants affect health. These are mediated by factors such as climate change and human-mediated events like pollution. Conversely, good design of cities—enhancing exercise and safety, for example—can create health-inducing environments.

Despite the obvious importance of public health and broad social, economic, and environmental impacts on the health of a nation, we will mostly focus in this workbook on designing changes in the organization, financing and delivery of individual healthcare services. We have chosen to emphasize individual healthcare services because of its importance to national economies, high costs, popularity, and political prominence, and, as we will argue, its unstoppable expansion and opportunity costs if medical care cannot be redesigned and improved.

Health, Economic Growth, and Development

The relationship between health and the economy is a two-way street. On the one hand, the interaction of health and the economy can be a virtuous cycle (Figure 1.2). A strong economy is a powerful predictor of good health. Economic growth, with the right policies, enhances health; individual health improves as socioeconomic status rises, A robust economy enables countries to invest in health systems that play important roles in improving health and social well-being of individuals and populations.

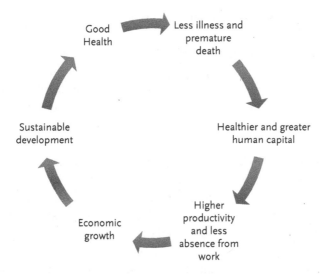

Figure 1.2 Health, economic growth, and development.

In addition to its benefits for individuals, families, and communities, health is a critical ingredient supporting economic growth and sustainable development of countries. Better health contributes to economic growth by producing healthy and productive human capital. The prospect of better health and longer lives incentivizes people to invest more in developing their human and social capital. Because healthy citizens have better chances to realize future benefits in employment and income, they are willing to commit upfront to more years of schooling for themselves and their children. For children, good health translates into high attendance at school and superior cognitive functioning. For adults, good health means less absence from work and greater ability to fulfill work duties, leading to higher productivity.

On the other hand, health and the economy can interact in a vicious cycle. A struggling economy can increase poverty and illness. Poor health leads to further reduced productivity and loss of human capital. These factors then hinder economic growth and produce more poverty, which in turn drives ill health, creating a vicious cycle. Moreover, the surge of illness can strain healthcare delivery and raise costs, sapping the economy of investments needed to recover from the economic downturn. Until they can control the costs of medical care, nations will have less available for other national priorities, including public health and stimulating economic growth.

It is self-evident that a high-performing health system should deliver value-for-money. It should generate the greatest possible health of its population for whatever financial inputs it dedicates to health. Well-functioning health systems use available resources efficiently and effectively to produce good health. They respond to legitimate expectations of citizens and satisfy them.

But what is *good health*? How would one know that their country achieved it? Measuring the health of a nation is complicated. Generic definitions of health vary widely, ranging from the idealistic aspirations of the World Health Organization (WHO) charter, which states "health is a state of complete physical, mental and social well-being and not merely the absence of disease or infirmity"[1] to the more modest and conditional definition expressed as the vision of the US Healthy People 2030 Framework that health is "a society in which all people can achieve their full potential for health and well-being across the lifespan."[2]

A high-performing health system and good health, as an expectation and objective of a nation, are in the eye of the beholder. Each nation has its own idea of good health. Beyond the general use of longevity as a measure of good health, countries differ in what they want to get from their health system. What a country wants in the way of good health and what it is willing to give up to achieve it reflect unique priorities. Understanding what an individual nation views as good health is key to assessing how well the output of their health system is doing the job.

Health is deeply intertwined with other factors that influence what citizens want and expect from their nation. Individuals want to live free of disease, disability, and death. But they also want to be safe, sheltered, and fed. Health systems are important for the productive economy and security of countries. Well-functioning health systems are critical in mounting effective responses to emerging public health emergencies, such as epidemics and pandemics from infectious diseases,[3] and in addressing burden of disease from other conditions, such as noncommunicable diseases and cancers.[4]

In practice, linking performance of health systems directly to good health has been challenging.[5] Many well-intentioned policies and managerial decisions aimed at improving health systems do not achieve desired outcomes and instead lead to unexpected or unintended consequences. One explanation for this phenomenon is that too often the tools used to conceptualize and analyze health systems and the heuristics used to generate managerial decisions are too simplistic for health systems that are complex. As a result, decision makers have limited understandings of how best to design a health system and translate it into policy.[6]

Several obvious factors influence the ways in which a country achieves good health efficiently, effectively, and equitably. The health system success factors include, among others, a vision for what they country wants, an excellent design of structures and processes in their health system, the capacity of individuals to make appropriate decisions in relation to their health, good management of healthcare institutions, and effective political leadership. These factors are influenced by contextual characteristics of the setting in which a country is situated, such as history of the country, sociocultural norms, economic characteristics, ability to introduce and scale up new technologies, and good doctors and hospitals.

SYSTEMS THINKING AND THE HEALTH SYSTEMS

The Evolution to a Systems Thinking Model for Health

Defining and describing a health system is difficult. A system is a collection of interacting elements that produce outputs that lead to outcomes. A system's elements hang together as a whole because they are linked, continually interact and affect each other and operate toward a common purpose.

A health system is a *means to an end*—a collection of activities designed to achieve societal goals. In simplistic terms, a health system uses inputs (money and other resources) to build and operate institutions that deliver healthcare services with structural and process characteristics that produce results that aim to meet citizen expectations about maintaining health, overcoming disease and illness, alleviating suffering, enhancing well-being, supporting shared national values, and creating good value-for-money.

Early attempts to conceptualize health systems described them in terms of the actors within them, economic relationships among the participants, or flows of funds. As an example of the first, systems were defined in terms of the main sets of actors needed for the population to be served: healthcare providers, third-party payers, and government as regulator.[7]

Later, a health system was conceived of as the economic relationship between demand, supply, and intermediary agencies that influence the supply–demand relationship.[8,9] The demand side refers to individuals, households, and populations whose actions influence health outcomes, and the supply side to institutions that produce the human and material resources to provide healthcare. The agencies refer to the state or government institutions responsible for financing, regulation, and purchasing of healthcare and other institutional purchasers (such as private insurers, public insurance funds, district health authorities, and health maintenance organizations).

Others have defined health systems in terms of archetypes of financing and healthcare delivery models.[10] In this formulation, a health system is characterized as a set of relationships between an array of components (financing, macro-organization of provision, payments, regulations, and persuasion [of behavior], referred to as *control knobs*[11]) or as a set of *functions*[12] that can be modified by policymakers to achieve health system goals.

Descriptions of health systems have expanded upon these three definitions. The WHO in 2000, for example, described a health system as comprising all the activities whose primary purpose is to promote, restore or maintain health.[13] They extended this definition in 2007 to include the people, institutions, and resources engaged in a variety of activities in accordance with established policies to improve the health of the population they serve, while responding to people's legitimate expectations and protecting them against the cost of ill-health.[14]

Most recently, however, health systems have come to be viewed as complex systems shaped by interacting functions, dynamic complexity, and contextual factors distinctive to each country.[15]

This way of describing a health system has been named *systems thinking* and is the approach we use in this workbook.

From Static Description to Dynamic Formulation

The daunting job of understanding systems is complicated by the way people try to portray them. Over the years, many theories and tools, ranging from relatively simple to complex, have been developed to describe, understand, and inform actions in systems.

One way to view a system is mechanistically, describing it primarily in terms of the types and number of variables involved and their cause–effect connections. Peter Senge, in his book *The Fifth Discipline*, calls this *detail complexity*.[16] The tools used to understand and take action from this systems perspective are familiar to designers—identifying elements and processes, mapping and diagramming them, analyzing their connections and flow, and redesigning the elements and their relationships. Such tools are built on the notion of cause–effect relationships between and among the system's variables.

In problems displaying straightforward detail complexity, cause–effect models can be simple and effective. In general, these problems are characterized not only by a manageable number of variables, but they are also comparatively free of personal interactions, disparate aims, conflicts of interests, differences in mental maps, and know-how among the participants.

However, some systems, such as health systems, are dynamic and complex. They are made up of many interconnected and interdependent elements that form extensive networks of feedback loops with time delays and nonlinear relationships. A system's activity is the result of the influence of one element on another through feedback. This interconnectedness and these interactions mean that a *system response* to a stimulus, perturbation, or intervention occurs as a result of the interactions between the system's elements, rather than the result of a change in one component.

With higher levels of detail complexity, simple analysis and decision-making often fail. The human mind takes shortcuts and makes errors, of which individuals are often unaware. When faced with configural problems, the human brain, in most cases, resorts to linear decision-making models. In such systems, the limits to information processing capability of the human mind means that feedback structures, nonlinearities, and the time-delays between actions and their consequences are ignored by tools designed for simple detail complexity. Faced with too many variables, we first make assumptions that reduce the amount of information used in understanding a situation. However, by simplifying mental cause–effect maps, ignoring time delays and feedback loops, and assuming there are no interpersonal conflicts and misunderstandings between actors in the system, analysts usually generate static options when making decisions. Senge concludes that this simplifying and reductionist approach "create(s) a snapshot showing how the system works at a moment in time."[17p31]

Making so many simplifying assumptions leads to explanatory conclusions or modeling that have such a high uncertainty or error that the answers are as likely to be wrong as right. Using such reductionist and linear approaches in decision-making in health systems creates *bounded rationality*.[18] This term refers to explanatory cause–effect models that fail to provide an accurate representation of the real world because they ignore possible wider impacts of policies and decisions, as well as unintended consequences of policies. Such simplistic analyses miss or overlook important sources of the problem. This leads to *misperception of feedback*, so that even when such information is available, consequences of interactions cannot be deduced rapidly and correctly. In such instances, inadequately considered interventions aimed at eliminating the problems do not produce expected results but lead to further unintended consequences and produce *policy resistance*.[19,20]

Senge defines a second type of system complexity.[17] He calls this *dynamic complexity*, where cause and effect are subtle and where the effects over time of interventions are not obvious. Conventional forecasting, planning and analysis methods are not equipped to deal with dynamic complexity.[17] The perspective needed to understand, design, and take action in systems with dynamic complexity is called *systems thinking*.

What Is Systems Thinking?

Systems thinking is a way of describing and thinking about a system. There are patterns of interrelationships between key components of the system. These interactions operate over time. Systems thinking is a tool to understand such a complex system. Its basis is a type of analytic frame called *systems theory*, which was invented a century ago to enable designers to understand a system in dynamic motion, rather than merely as a set of component parts. Systems thinking is a way of thinking about the forces and inter-relationships that shape the behavior of systems.[17]

The essence of systems thinking is a way of looking that facilitates understanding the interconnectedness and behavior that characterizes the system as a whole rather than its individual component parts. With systems thinking, a designer can visualize patterns of change in systems and their movement over time, rather than as *static snapshots*.[16] It is akin to watching a video that shows all the moving parts of a system while they are in dynamic action producing their outputs.

Systems Thinking Is Needed to Understand Health Systems

Why is a systems approach necessary in improving health? Decision-making in health systems is characterized by *detail complexity*. To understand systems, a designer decision maker must have a way to understand its moving parts, interactions, interdependencies, timing delays, external influences, and feedback from outside the boundaries of the system itself. For simple systems, linear flow models offer easy ways to characterize inputs, structures and processes, and outputs. As systems increase in complexity, such models no longer suffice. They suffer from the limits of information processing capability of the human mind, which adapts to complexity by reducing the amount of information used, creating simple cause–effect mental maps, and generating a number of static options when making decisions. This limitation means that feedback structures, nonlinearities in systems, and the delays between actions and their consequences are ignored.

A functioning health *system* is more than the sum of its parts; it is a collection of stakeholders that form moving parts in a dynamic, interacting process. Systems thinking reveals the dynamic complexity of systems that are characterized by networks of relations, feedback loops, and nonlinearity.[21] Systems thinking fosters *the ability to see the world as a complex system* comprising many interconnected and interdependent parts.[22] It encourages looking at organizational dynamics and the interrelationships in the system, instead of getting overinvolved in the details of a situation. It helps anticipate rather than react to events and thus to prepare better for emerging challenges.

Dynamic complexity has important policy implications for health systems. If a health system's complexities are not understood, its policies may not lead to intended results and may even produce results that are counterintuitive or even the opposite of what was intended. One has to consider the effects of a policy not just on a component part but also on the system as a whole and anticipate the *system's response*.

Introduction to Health Systems

A health system is a system in a special sense of the word. When we use the term *system* in this workbook, we mean it as a general descriptive term that refers to the way that an enterprise functions as a whole. *Systems* are a collection of elements interacting and joined together by a web of interrelationships. What a system produces is the result of the workings of its design, elements, people, processes, interconnections, and interactions. All its outputs are latent in the structure of the system. It is an interactive collection of activities whose design determines—and even predetermines—its behavior. In other words, systems generate their own behavior.

Every enterprise is a system with a structure organized according to a set of principles and rules. Systems produce something. Each system is designed to produce the results it gets; its performance potential is determined by its design and structure, while its actual outputs are further modified by its level of efficiency and effectiveness. Using a common example, imagine a racing car that has a potential top speed of 170 miles per hour. This speed is achievable because of the design of the car, its motor, its drivetrain, and other structural features. To achieve its full potential performance, however, it needs a skilled driver who must be effective—that is, doing all the right things in steering, braking, and throttling up and down—and it must be efficient: potential performance is lost when parts are worn, the transmission does not work efficiently, and tuning is not optimal.

Like all systems, health systems are built in such a way that its underlying structure determines how it generates and expresses its results; the health system releases its performance in a way that is latent in its structure. Someone designed parts of it, science advanced its capacities, and it evolved through many large and small iterations to its current complex set of people, processes, and things.

Systems Thinking and Systems Theory to the Rescue

Systems thinking is a discipline that consists of broad concepts that help one to understand and characterize systems that experience dynamic complexity (and higher levels of detail complexity as well). Systems thinking is a framework for seeing interrelationships and repeated events rather than a specific activity, for seeing patterns of change, and for considering human behavior within systems and over time. It facilitates an understanding of organizational dynamics and the interrelationships in the system, instead of getting bogged down in the mechanical details of a situation.

In systems thinking, an organization and its respective context is viewed as a complex whole. The core of systems thinking is the ability to see the world as a complex system, comprising many interconnected and interdependent parts.[22] It enables an observer to see the whole as well as its component parts: simultaneously seeing the tree and the woods, so to speak. Understanding interconnectedness and complexity is the essence of systems thinking.

Systems theory, on which systems thinking is based, originated in the 1920s within several disciplines, including biology and engineering, as a response to growing technological complexities that confronted engineering and science. It evolved further with the field of system dynamics, developed in 1950s by Jay Forrester at the Massachusetts Institute of Technology, who recognized the need for better methods of testing new ideas in social systems.[23]

In practice, systems thinking entails careful consideration of possible consequences of policies and actions. This involves generation of scenarios through group work and joint thinking and discussing the possible implications of each scenario. Finding ways to mitigate unintended consequences of polices or interventions—taking into account interactions between health system elements and its context—is also an essential component of systems thinking.

Systems thinking can help overcome the limitations of linear and reductionist approaches in policymaking by enabling testing of new ideas in social systems.[23] In practice, shifting to systems thinking means considering the interlinkages between system elements and the interactions between the systems and the context within which the system is situated. One has to consider the effects of a policy, not just on a component part but also on the environment as a whole and anticipate the *context's response*. This places greater emphasis on fostering collaboration, careful thinking through of possible consequences of actions, and generating scenarios through group working.

Systems thinking involves collaboration across disciplines, sectors, and organizations with ongoing learning that recognizes that the context and health system interactions are continuously changing, and that policymakers need to adapt, learn, and apply new knowledge to evolving challenges. It considers organizational structures, patterns of interaction, and events as components of larger structures, helping to anticipate rather than react to events, which in turns allows policymakers to better prepare for emerging challenges.

Health Systems and Systems Thinking

A health system is no different than other complex dynamic systems. A health system evolved as a response to an immediate threat or to fulfill societal or political ambitions (e.g., the development of the Bismarck model of health systems that established welfare systems in Prussia and central Europe or the predominantly tax-funded national health systems as characterized by the United Kingdom (UK) and Nordic countries in Europe). The resulting health system responded by producing outputs: health, relief from the effects of illness, reassurance, satisfaction, and hope.

Complex systems can only be changed by understanding their internal dynamics and making targeted interventions at high leverage points that catalyze transformative change. It is the first objective of organizations and systems to achieve the inherent capacity of the system's design by improving efficiency and effectiveness through design and management. In general, efficiency is achieved through understanding and modifying feedback loops internal to the system. Effectiveness, on the other hand, depends also on feedback from, understanding of, and adjustment to the context external to the system. When the limits of improvements from efficiency and effectiveness are reached, the relative cost of managing inputs and delivering results begins to rise, and when this point is reached in a system, it is time to improve the system's inherent capacity to produce outputs that make it more effective in achieving its desired outcomes and goals.

CHAPTER 2

Assessing the Health System of a Country

Chapter 2 presents an approach to understanding and analyzing health systems. The chapter is structured as a teaching plan and workbook. First, it presents a health system analytic framework (Figure 2.1) that will be used throughout the book. Each of the model's elements is explained, and suggestions made about what is included and how observational data for these elements can be found. Second, following the introduction of this framework, we describe how the model will be used as the basis of a student's independent study of one country that they select for their work during the course.

After working independently, students will break into groups of four to six and will meet for about two hours (in person or virtually) to discuss and analyze contextual factors and how they are changing and how these changes are creating opportunities for and threats to health systems. The groups will then undertake another period of independent study to characterize functions of the country's existing health system, the health service outputs it produces, and national goals. This study will be followed by another small team exercise, in which each group will use the framework for health system analysis described later in the chapter to analyze this second tranche of information about their chosen country (although the model can be applied to any population with its own healthcare program, such as a union, a military veterans' system, or a large business). The group will also formulate a presentation of their conclusions.

This chapter's teaching and learning plan, which may take two to three weeks to complete, ideally culminates in a whole-course group meeting, where each subgroup presents their analysis to other students and faculty for comment and

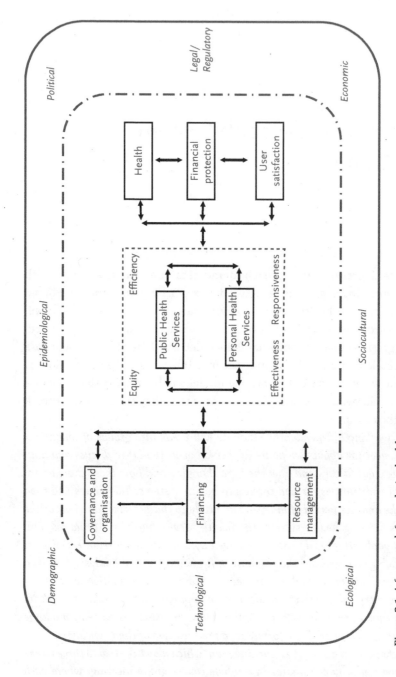

Figure 2.1 A framework for analyzing health systems.

Source: Atun R, Aydin S, Chakraborty S, et al. Universal health coverage in Turkey: enhancement of equity. *Lancet.* 2013;382(9886):65–99; supplementary appendix: http://download.thelancet.com/mmcs/journals/lancet/PIIS014067361361051X/mmc1.pdf?id=eaa9nRX05fcXdhZf5ODCu

critique. The presentation, which should be written up in summary form, will cover the context of the country studied, the organizational design and governance of the health system, how resources are managed, how the health system is financed, major features of its healthcare delivery, performance of the health systems, and one policy or structural change the country has undertaken. The presenting group will identify and describe its first impressions of any major shortfalls in achieving health system goals and will present its preliminary view of the gaps in health systems achievements in relation to outcomes or outputs, and their impact on the health and well-being of the population.

HEALTH SYSTEMS: DEFINITIONS AND CONCEPTUALIZATIONS

A health system is a means to an end—a system designed to achieve societal goals regarding health and well-being. Recent definitions, such as that by the World Health Organization (WHO) in 2000, describe a health system as all the activities whose primary purpose is to promote, restore, or maintain health.[1] The WHO extended this definition in 2007 to include the people, institutions, and resources, arranged together in accordance with established policies, to improve the health of the population they serve, while responding to people's legitimate expectations and protecting them against the cost of ill health through a variety of activities whose primary intent is to improve health.[2]

Earlier definitions conceptualized and described health systems from a specific viewpoint. These have included descriptions from the perspective of the range of actors within them, economic relationships, or flows of funds. For example, Evans defined health systems in terms of the main sets of actors comprising the population to be served: healthcare providers, third-party payers, and government as regulator.[3]

Others have described a health system in terms of the economic relationship between demand, supply, and intermediary agencies that influence the supply–demand relationship. The demand side refers to individuals, households, and populations whose actions drive the choices and outcomes of health services and outcomes. The supply side denotes the institutions that produce human and material resources for healthcare, providers of healthcare services, individuals, and informal unpaid carers. The agencies refer to the state or government institutions responsible for financing, regulation, and purchasing of healthcare and other institutional purchasers (such as private insurers, public insurance funds, district health authorities, and health maintenance organizations).[4]

Others have defined health systems in terms of archetypes of financing and delivery of healthcare, describing them as an array of relationships between a set of components such as financing, macro-organization of provision, payments, regulations, and persuasion (of behavior). The components have been named by Roberts and others as control knobs[5] and by Frenk as a set of functions[6] that can be modified by policymakers to achieve health system goals.

More recently, health systems have been conceptualized as complex systems characterized by interacting functions and dynamic complexity and shaped by contextual factors in each country.[7] This way of describing a health system is called *systems thinking* and is the approach we use in this workbook (see Box 2.1).

Box 2.1: USING SYSTEMS THINKING TO UNDERSTAND HEALTH SYSTEMS AS COMPLEX SYSTEMS

For simple systems, flow models offer easy ways to characterize inputs, structures and processes, and outputs. Such flow diagrams are like snapshots of the parts of a system. As systems increase in complexity, such models no longer suffice. They suffer from the limits of information processing capability of the human mind, which adapts to complexity by reducing the amount of information used, creating simple cause–effect mental maps, and generating a number of static options when making decisions. This limitation means that feedback structures, nonlinearities in systems, and the delays between actions and their consequences are ignored.

Decision-making in health systems is characterized by detail complexity. To understand systems, a designer decision maker must have a way to understand its moving parts, interactions, interdependencies, timing delays, external influences, and feedback from outside the boundaries of the system itself.

Systems thinking is a tool to understand a complex system. Its basis is a type of analytic frame called *systems theory*, which was invented a century ago to enable designers to understand a system in dynamic motion, rather than merely as a set of component parts. Systems thinking is "a way of thinking about, and a language for describing and understanding, the forces and inter-relationships that shape the behavior of systems."[8p6] The essence of systems thinking is a way of looking that facilitates understanding the interconnectedness and behavior that characterizes the system as a whole rather than its individual component parts. With systems thinking, a designer can visualize patterns of change in systems and

---

their movement over time, rather than as static snapshots.[9] It is akin to watching a video that shows all the moving parts of a system while they are in dynamic action producing their outputs.

System thinking reveals the dynamic complexity of systems that are characterized by networks of relations, feedback loops, and nonlinearity. Systems thinking enables one to see the world as a complex system that consists of many interconnected and interdependent parts.[10] It encourages looking at organizational dynamics and the interrelationships in the system, instead of getting overinvolved in the details of a situation. It helps anticipate rather than react to events and thus to prepare better for emerging challenges.

Dynamic complexity has important policy implications for health systems. If a health system's complexities are not understood, its policies may not lead to intended results and may even produce results that are the opposite of what was intended. One has to consider the effects of a policy not just on a component part but also on the system as a whole and anticipate the system's response.

FRAMEWORK FOR CONCEPTUALIZING AND ANALYZING HEALTH SYSTEMS

We have developed a holistic framework (Figure 2.1) that extends earlier approaches used to analyze health systems[11,12] by adopting a *systems view of health systems* and in incorporating *context* as an integral part of an all-encompassing analysis.[13] In this view, health systems are conceptualized as comprising a set of interlinked functions: (i) governance and organization, (ii) financing, and (iii) resource generation and management. These functions can be modified by policies and interact in a dynamic way to produce a set of outputs in the form of public health and personal healthcare services for citizens. Public health and healthcare services operate with varied levels of effectiveness, efficiency, equity, and responsiveness to achieve health system outcomes of health, financial protection, and user satisfaction. The nature and functioning of the health system, and the outputs and outcomes it produces, are shaped by the context within which the system is situated and with which it interacts in a dynamic fashion.[14,15]

Using this systems perspective, one can explore contextual factors and health systems functions that interact to influence health system performance and the achievement of health system goals and objectives. The model conceptualizes health systems as comprising a set of interlinked functions (governance and organization, financing, resource generation and management), which operate in a contextual milieu and produce a range of outputs. Those functions, and the structural design in which they operate, can be modified by policies. They also interact in a dynamic manner to produce a set of outputs in the form of public health and personal health-care services for citizens, with varied levels of effectiveness, efficiency, equity, and responsiveness. These outputs, in turn, produce population-level outcomes of health, financial protection, and user satisfaction.

The framework used in this chapter can be used to understand and examine how a health system works. It enables analysis of health systems from contextual factors affecting health system functions to health system outputs (public health and personal health service delivery) and outcomes (population health, financial protection and user satisfaction). This framework can also be used as a tool to analyze a health system's performance, as an evaluative instrument to assess effects of enacted policies or changes in health system functions, or as a formative tool to develop and test future policies or scenarios. The analytical framework has been used in single-country and multicountry analyses and to inform health system reforms.[16]

Individual Assignment

Each student should pick a country from the following list. The best choice will blend three criteria: a country with which you are familiar, one that you are especially interested in learning about, and a country that you share with at least one other small group of students. You will still have an opportunity to switch your choice after the small group meeting, coming up next in this chapter. The country choices are*

- *Brazil*
- *Germany*
- *South Africa*
- *South Korea*
- *The Netherlands*
- *Turkey*
- *United Kingdom*
- *United States of America*

Prior to the first small group meeting, each student will work independently to apply the framework to the country of their choice. Table 2.1 provides a format for keeping track of your observations and initial impressions. As you apply the framework to your selected country, your first impressions of its strengths and problems are useful. Use Table 2.1 as instructed to make notes prior to the small

Table 2.1 FORMAT FOR RECORDING COUNTRY ANALYSIS AND INITIAL IMPRESSIONS

	Notes	Impressions of Strengths and Weaknesses
Context		
D		
E		
P		
L		
E		
S		
E		
T		
Functions		
Governance/organization		
Financing		
Resource management		
Objectives		
Equity		
Efficiency		
Effectiveness		
Responsiveness		
Goals		
Health		
Financial Protection		
National satisfaction		

Context abbreviations, in order: D, demographic; E, epidemiological; P, political; L, legal and regulatory; E, economic; S, sociocultural; E, ecological, T, technological *group meeting. You will return to this chart, or a copy, at several points in later chapters.*

Context

When introducing health system reforms, the context of the existing health system is vitally important for reformers, policymakers, and change-makers to consider. Even when there is ample evidence of the benefits of a policy or an intervention, contextual factors influence these policies and affect their introduction and scale-up. Specifically, analysis and understanding of context can help provide legitimacy to new policies, reveal important historical antecedents, offer insight into political systems, and provide an understanding of the influence of sociocultural norms (which affect cognitive and normative legitimacy of policies). Technological innovations (such as digital social media for mass communication) can create new possibilities for interventions into health systems and influence the introduction and scale-up of policies. Critical events (such as regime change in governments, economic crisis, rapid economic growth, natural disasters, and epidemics) create external shocks on health systems that may facilitate or hamper change.

In our framework, we define context in terms of factors that individually and through their interactions influence the trajectory of change in health systems for better or for worse. For example, ecological changes can lead to adverse health effects from generation of environments conducive to emergence of new infections, floods, heatwaves, water shortage, landslides, and exposure to ultraviolet radiation or pollutants. Ecological changes can also lead to ecosystem-mediated health effects such as altered infectious disease risk (e.g., emergence of zoonoses—infectious diseases that are transmissible from animals to humans through direct contact or though food, water, and the environment), reduced food yields that lead to undernutrition and stunting, depletion of natural medicines, and worsening mental health. Further, ecological changes can produce indirect health effects such as those due to population displacement from injudicious deforestation, conflict, and forced migration.

Some contextual factors are facilitators of positive change. As an example, technological changes create major opportunities for health systems to achieve systems goals and objectives. For example, digital data have made it possible to collect large amounts of clinical, socioeconomic, demographic, lifestyle, health behavior, and genetic data on individuals and populations and to create large data sets from such multiple sources.

It has also facilitated new communication technologies that transfer and pool these data in large databases. Advances in fast-computing, data science, artificial intelligence, and machine learning and the development of new investigational and evaluative methods have made possible the analysis of large amounts of data. Using these novel analytic approaches, analysis of such information makes it possible to identify which individuals in different populations are at greater risk of developing certain illnesses, to estimate potential benefit of interventions, and to compute relative risk of death from certain diseases with or without an intervention. The ability to analyze such large data sets to identify individual characteristics and their propensity to illness or death has enabled risk stratification and classification of individuals or population groups into risk categories. Risk stratification of individuals or population groups and information about their ability to benefit from an intervention has enabled the development of *precision medicine* for individuals and *precision health* for populations, both of which offer the opportunity to precisely target treatments and interventions.

The interplay of contextual factors influences the trajectory of change in health systems and delineates what change seems possible. Changes in each contextual factor and major contextual shifts—which can create external shocks—and their interplay create *opportunities* or *threats* for health systems in the short- or long-term to influence its performance, outputs, and outcomes. The analysis of context can identify opportunities that are conducive to attaining desired health system goals and objectives in line with the values embraced by stakeholders. In relation to threats, the analysis can identify contextual changes that may hinder the attainment of desired health system outcomes or may worsen health system performance.

As you consider the different contextual elements of your chosen country's health system, you should be identifying and weighing their impact on the health system. Your analysis will seek to identify and map contextual factors to ascertain which of the changes create opportunities and which create threats to the health system now and in the future. Analyzing your country's context aims to answer six questions:

1. What are the most important changes, positive or negative, among the eight context categories?
2. How are these changes affecting the health system?
3. What is the likely magnitude of these changes on the health system?
4. How and when will these changes impact the health system?
5. How certain is the likely impact?
6. Which of these changes create opportunities and which create threats to the health system?

Table 2.2 COVID-19—THE INTERPLAY OF CONTEXT AND HEALTH SYSTEMS

Context	Contextual Changes
Demographic	Aging—vulnerable populations with multimorbidity
Epidemiological	Emerging infections SARS-CoV-2 and climate change's effect on disease vectors
Political	Leadership and attitudes toward command and control
Legal	The delays from existing rules and regulations at a time of national urgency
Economic	Globalization—interdependence and supply chains' impact on world economy and trade of good and services
Sociocultural norms	Attitudes toward death and dying and the value of intensive medicine for the old and frail
Ecological changes	Destruction of animal natural habitats—leading to mixing of human and animal ecosystems—emergence of new infections (e.g., coronaviruses)
Technology	Travel; digital data; data analysis and modeling; social media; communications; new diagnostics; technology-enabled testing and tracing systems; integrated supply chains

In our framework, we define context by a set of descriptive categories that are continually changing and influencing each other. These factors include demographic, epidemiological, political, legal and regulatory, economic, sociocultural, ecological, and technological factors. Changes in these contextual factors strongly affect health systems. In turn, performance of health systems influences the context. See Table 2.2 for an illustrative example of how changes in context shape health systems and how health system responses to these changes shape context in different countries.

Context Categories

We discuss in more detail each of the contextual factors in our framework with a series of questions aimed at assessing the contextual factor. Table 2.3 summarizes key descriptive parameters and some suggested available measurements to estimate contextual factors.

Table 2.3 KEY DESCRIPTIVE PARAMETERS AND EXAMPLES
OF CONTEXTUAL FACTORS

Contextual Factors	Descriptive Parameters	Examples of Parameters Used
Demographic	Population dynamics: population growth and structure	• Aging • Migration • Urbanization
Epidemiological	Trends for risk, morbidity, and mortality	• Noncommunicable diseases • Multimorbidity • Emerging infections
Political	Political economy Institutional configuration Citizen engagement	• Government values • Government stability • Civil society role in decision-making and accountability
Legal and regulatory	International agreements National laws	• Trade agreements
Economic	Economic growth Favorability of economic environment	• Fiscal space • Gross domestic product growth • Unemployment levels • Inflation trends
Sociocultural	Public attitudes and beliefs related to health Social norms Lifestyles	• Citizen values and expectations • Social networks
Ecological	Human and urban ecology Physical environment	• Natural disasters • Climate change
Technological	Technologies for health and health technologies	• Technological adoption (communication, computing, data science)

Demographics

Demographic characterization refers to the status and trends in age structure, gender, and geographic distribution of the population. Demographic patterns can be stable or vary over time, in relation to factors such as fertility, mortality, immigration, and migration. For example, the speed and extent of demographic transition reflects the dynamics between changes in population, fertility, and mortality levels in a country. Demographic transition in a country occurs with a decline in mortality rates, followed—after a lag—by a reduction in total fertility rate, bringing about an initial transitional period of high population growth (as more children and adults survive and live longer) before fertility levels adjust to longer life span and the population stabilizes. With demographic transition, increased longevity and reduced total fertility cause a swing in the population age profile, leading to a shift toward an aging population and a declining proportion of younger and working age individuals.

Key Questions

> How does the nation's demographic profile affect the health system?
> How are the general population dynamics changing in the country of analysis in relation to infant mortality rate and total fertility rate?
> How are the general population dynamics changing in relation to average life expectancy at birth, population age structure, and population size?
> What are the levels of urban and rural populations? What are the urbanization trends?
> What are the trends in relation to immigration and emigration in and out of the country?
> What are the implications of the demographic transition on the health system?

Epidemiological Factors

Epidemiological factors refer to the pattern of health and disease in the country. An epidemiologic transition typically follows a demographic transition; falling mortality and fertility level and increased longevity lead to an aging population and consequent change in the population age structure.

Epidemiologic transition creates new patterns of risk factors, illness, and causes of death. Patterns dominated by infectious diseases and conditions affecting children and pregnant women shift to those in which chronic diseases, cancer, and mental health conditions increasingly predominate. Demographic and epidemiological transitions bring about major changes in population age structure and the burden of disease, and the stage countries are in during these transitions will determine the types of policies needed to improve health and benefit countries economically and socially.

What is the epidemiologic profile of the nation and how does it impact the country and its health system?

How is the epidemiologic profile changing?

How are mortality levels changing in the population and population subsegments (infant mortality, maternal mortality, mortality levels of major chronic diseases)?

Which conditions are rising or falling in incidence or prevalence (for key noncommunicable and communicable diseases)?

How is the prevalence of risk factors for chronic diseases changing (e.g., smoking and obesity) in the population or in population groups?

How are social determinants of health changing in the population or in population subgroups?

Political Environment

These characteristics describe the inclusiveness, continuity, effectiveness, and values of government. Features include political stability, government structures, and political inclusion of citizens and civil society. The political environment also relates, among others, to the political economy in terms of decisions related to health. Politics in a country reveals the prevailing values of the citizens and government that shape societal goals and broad policy objectives, especially those related to social sectors. The political environment delimits readiness for change.

Key Questions

How effective and stable is the political environment?

How trusted is the government's leadership?

Who makes political decisions?

What are the values of the government?

How do these values influence policies on health?

What is the balance of power between the executive, legislative, and judiciary?

How does this balance influence the decision-making process in the country in relation to health?

How important is health as an issue for politicians?

What is the capacity of the political system for innovation and change in health systems?

At what level are decisions affecting health made (e.g., national, state, province, municipality, city, institution)?

Legal and Regulatory Environment

These factors describe the national or international legal and regulatory rules (beyond those health polices or regulations that directly guide the activities in the health system) that constrain or support the structure, function, and financing of health systems. These include, for example, data privacy laws, binding international legal agreements in areas such as climate change, international accords governing human rights, international treaties governing trade (such as, for example, the World Trade Organization), bilateral trade agreements, and multicountry or regional trade agreements.

Key Questions

What important laws of the country affect the health system (e.g., laws on data privacy, anticompetitive marketplace interference, and workforce accreditation)?

What international treaties to which the country is signatory are likely to affect the health system or health policies (e.g., the United Nations' treaties on human rights, the Framework Convention on Tobacco Control, treaties governing the World Trade Organization)?

What bilateral, multicountry, or regional trade agreements has the country entered into that may affect health?

Economy

Economic factors relate to the economic strength of a country—including economic policies, economic growth, economic stability, economic sustainability, and the way that individuals and businesses benefit from the current economy and its success and weakness.

What is the economic outlook (e.g., economic growth trends as measured by changes in gross domestic product, government debt levels, current account balance, employment levels, and inflation level)?

What are the levels and trends of income distribution, wealth, and poverty?

How progressive is the income distribution and upward mobility, comparatively speaking?

What is the likely impact of the economic environment on individuals, households, and communities and their behavior in relation to health?

What are the effects of economic trends on social determinants of health?

What is the likely impact of the economic environment on the government's fiscal capacity for allocations to the public sector health budget; what are the prospects for private sector investment?

What is the economic environment for financial investment in innovation and development in healthcare delivery and medical technologies such as devices, drugs, and different service delivery modalities?

Sociocultural Dynamics

Sociocultural dynamics relate to global sentiments, values, attitudes, expectations, and beliefs among the population, especially as they relate to health and healthcare. Included are general social attitudes about medical care as a right, individual freedom versus social solidarity, and the value and importance of medical care. Among the most important of values and expectations of citizens are those affecting care-seeking (i.e., stiff upper lip vs. care-seeking) and following medical care advice; lifestyle and behavioral choices of citizens (e.g., tobacco use, diet, and physical activity); adherence to advice; risk perceptions (fatalistic versus opportunistic, tolerance of discomfort and anxiety); cultural norms (such as beliefs about shamans, causality of disease from curses or punishment, traditional medicine); class systems; and gender norms.

Key Questions

What are the prevailing sociocultural norms in relation to health?

What are the prevailing sociocultural norms in relation to social determinants of health?

How do sociocultural norms and dynamics affect the health system and health policies?

What sociocultural practices are most likely to accelerate or retard change?

Ecological Changes

Ecological changes relate to the status of and changes in the physical and ecological environment affecting health. These include degradation, depletion, and destruction of natural systems that lead to, among others, loss in biodiversity, decline in availability of ice-free and desert-free surface land resources and natural forests, diminishing fresh water resources, increased salination of fresh water stores, rising amounts of liquid and solid waste that are not effectively managed, increased acidification of oceans, atmospheric aerosol loading, stratospheric ozone depletion, and, most concerning of all, global warming and climate change, which exacerbate these aforementioned changes.

Key Questions

What are the major ecological changes in the country?

What factors are driving these ecological changes?

What are the direct health effects of these changes?

What is the ecosystem-mediated health effects of these changes?

What are indirect, deferred, and displaced health effects of these changes?

Technological Changes

This category assesses the state of technology in the country, the rate and direction of technological developments that relate to advances shaping health systems and their adoption. Categories include, but are not limited to, scientific advances in life sciences (genetics, genomics, systems biology, cell biology), communication and information technologies, advances in computing and analytic methods, digitization of data, advances in data science, and improvements in geographic information systems and their application.

Many advances relate to technologies in other sectors that enable delivery of more efficient, effective, and responsive health services (communication, computing, data science, transport, environmental management, supply chain management systems) and health technologies (diagnostics, vaccines, medicines, clinical decision support, and medical devices). These technological advances in the health sector could be harnessed to enhance the resources available (medicines, diagnostics) and the provision of healthcare services.

Key Questions

How are major technological changes in your study country being used to improve the health system?

How widely are these technologies being used and what is their effect on the health system?

How are health technologies affecting healthcare service delivery, costs, and quality (directly or indirectly)?

How is technology affecting communication, integration, and coordination of care?

Small Group Exercise: Analyzing Context

Prior to the small group meeting, the course administrator or the teaching fellow should prepare the logistics. They should elicit each student's choice of a country to study, assign the group into work teams of about four to six students each, inform the students about their workgroup, and distribute contact information.

This small group exercise can be conducted virtually or in person and will last approximately two hours. This exercise is aimed at enabling the students to apply the following analytic framework to explore how key context factors are changing, to identify major trends and contextual shifts, and to ascertain how these shifts may impact the health system to create opportunities and threats. The objective is both to refine each student's understanding of contextual factors and to begin to shape among small group members a consensus on the contextual changes and major contextual shifts and how these changes and shifts are affecting health systems. This exercise will be followed by another period of self-study of the 10 other attributes of their health system.

The exercise consists of four steps, which are described next and should be undertaken as a team process. A single student should be assigned to take the lead in filling out each of the three tables. That person should lead the discussion of that section.

Step 1: Identification of Key Contextual Shifts (30 Minutes)

Ask the following questions to identify three important contextual changes and one major contextual shift. List them in Table 2.4 with the rationale for selecting a particular change as a major contextual shift.

Ask the following questions to inform your analysis:

1. How would you describe the contextual changes?
2. In your view, which one or two of these changes represent a major contextual shift?
3. Why do you think the change you have identified is a major contextual shift?

Step 2: Analyze the Nature of Contextual Changes, Their Potential Magnitude and the Timing of These Shifts (30 Minutes)

In this step you will continue your group work to identify the nature of the contextual shifts (e.g., rapid, one-off, or slow-incremental), the likely magnitude of the impact of these shifts on the health system, the timing of the impact, and the certainty of the shift and impact. Once you have answered the following questions, you can map your answers in Table 2.5.

Ask the following questions to inform your analysis:

1. What is the nature of the shift (one-off, rapid, or slow-incremental change)?
2. What is the likely magnitude of impact of these shifts on the health system?
3. Qualitatively estimate the level of impact as low-, medium- or high-impact (e.g., aging will lead to high increased chronic diseases and demand on health systems and is likely to be high-impact).

Table 2.4 IDENTIFYING CONTEXTUAL CHANGES AND KEY CONTEXTUAL SHIFTS

Contextual Factors	Changes	Major Shift	Rationale for Selecting the Change as a Major Contextual Shift
Demographic	1. 2. 3.		
Epidemiological	1. 2. 3.		
Political	1. 2. 3.		
Legal and Regulatory	1. 2. 3.		
Economic	1. 2. 3.		
Socio-cultural	1. 2. 3.		
Ecological	1. 2. 3.		
Technological	1. 2. 3.		

4. When will these shifts impact the health system? Estimate the likely timing of impact (short-term is 1–3 years, medium-term is 4–10 years, and long-term is >10 years).
5. How certain is the likely impact? Estimate the likelihood of change and impact. For example, aging is fairly certain, prolonged economic crises can be predicted with medium certainty, and earthquakes (unless you live near a geological fault) are low certainty, although they might have high impact.

Table 2.5 NATURE OF CONTEXTUAL SHIFTS, THEIR POTENTIAL MAGNITUDE AND THE TIMING OF THESE SHIFTS

Contextual Factor	Contextual Shift	Extent of Impact			Timing of Impact			Certainty of Change and Impact		
		Low	Med	High	Short Term	Medium Term	Long Term	Low	Medium	High
Demographic										
Epidemiological										
Political										
Legal and regulatory										
Economic										
Sociocultural										
Ecological										
Technological										

Step 3: Identify How These Changes Might Impact Your Health System, and Delineate the Opportunities or Threats These Changes Might Create (1 Hour)

In this step. the group will continue to analyze the potential effects of the consensus contextual shifts your group has identified. Outline, with flow diagrams, the causal steps and pathway showing how the shifts ultimately influence the health system and identify whether the consequent changes create opportunities, threats, or both.

Ask the following questions to inform your analysis:

1. How might this shift affect the health system (e.g., increased demand for services; widening inequalities; shortage of funding)?
2. Develop a logic model or a causal pathway to map how the change might impact the health system directly or indirectly.
3. Categorize the contextual shifts into opportunities and threats.

Step 4: Create a Positioning Map of Contextual Shifts in Terms of Strength of Impact on Health System, Anticipated Time of Impact, and Certainty of Change (30 Minutes)

Work in your subgroups to combine the analyses from Steps 1 to 3 and use Figure 2.2 to generate a map of major contextual shifts and the opportunities and threats they generate.

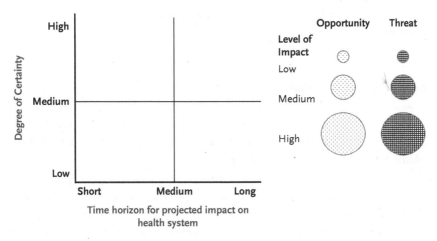

Figure 2.2 An at-a-glance map of opportunities and threats.

Individual Assignment

Proceeding from the first small group discussion of context, the students return to individual study of the remaining 10 descriptors of a generic health system. This section ends with another small group meeting during which their country analysis is finalized and readied for presentation in the culminating event of this chapter; that is, a large group meeting in which each subgroup presents its summary country analysis for review and comment.

Health System Functions

The framework identifies three major health system functions (governance and organization, financing, and resource management), which policymakers can modify to produce a set of desired health system outputs (personal health services and public health services) to reach targets designed to realize their policy objectives (effectiveness, efficiency, equity and responsiveness) and health system outcomes (health, financial protection, and user satisfaction).

The health system functions could be viewed as inputs to the system or as independent variables that policymakers can modify to achieve dependent health system objectives and outcomes. These functions are interdependent but modifiable variables that shape the structure and operations of the existing health system, facilitating or blocking change. Changing these functions is a big challenge because they interact with all other initiatives undertaken by governments on behalf of the populations they serve. Left in place, these functions may impede or facilitate change in health system. We discuss each of the three functions in turn.

Governance and Organization

Governance and organization relate to the structural and functional organization of the health system, particularly the institutional relationships within the health system, including

1. the organizational structure of public health and personal healthcare services, including the role of the ministry of health in relation to other actors in the health system such as insurers, purchasing organizations, and regulatory agencies;

2. the extent of geographic decentralization of decision-making (e.g., to states, provinces, districts, municipalities, or autonomous public healthcare institutions with independent boards);
3. extent of functional decentralization (the decision-making powers are devolved or delegated to geographic entities in respect of financing, planning, budgeting, service design, and management of physical and human resources);
4. the scope of regulation and competition in the health sector, which influences the extent of innovation, demand and supply patterns, and prices of services; and
5. the degree of public and private sector involvement in financing and provision of health services, and the extent to which they interact to effectively use available capacity and assets in the health system (Box 2.2).

Box 2.2: ORGANIZATION AND GOVERNANCE—
COUNTRY EXAMPLES

CANADA VERSUS UNITED STATES

There is geographic and functional decentralization of the health system. In both countries states (in the United States) and provinces (in Canada) have substantial major role in governance, financing, and resource management of the health system. However, the extent of regulation and competition in each country varies, and as a result, the extent of state involvement in the delivery of public health or personal health services. The United States has much higher degree of competition with many private insurers and independent healthcare providers, whereas in a neighboring country, Canada, there are no private insurers, far higher levels of regulation, limited competition, and healthcare providers are all part of a single, structured provincial public system.

As with the differences in organization and governance of health systems, the role of the ministries of health vary from country to country. Ministries may undertake these functions or devolve them to agencies (e.g., an insurance agency or a private insurer for financing or a quality agency to oversee quality monitoring and assessment).

Typically, ministries of health are responsible for the following.

1. Health system development
   • Policy development
   • Strategic planning

- Intersectoral collaboration
- Social mobilization
- Defining priorities and service packages

2. Health system coordination
   - Managing health system capacity
   - Deciding on the use of costly high technology
3. Design of health system financing
   - How priorities are set
   - How funds are allocated within the health system
4. Regulation
   - Sanitary—public health
   - Healthcare services—licensing, accreditation, certification
   - Quality assurance
   - Setting standards
5. Ensuring preparedness for major events and shocks, e.g.,
   - Epidemics
   - Natural disasters
   - Bioterrorism
6. Consumer protection
   - Protecting citizens' rights and ensuring their safety.

Key Questions

1. How are health policy decisions made—centrally or decentralized?
2. Does the country's governance favor regulatory approaches or market forces?
3. What do you see as the strengths and weaknesses of your country's organization and governance?

Financing

Financing function is concerned with where funding comes from and how it is applied. Variables include how funds are collected, how they are pooled, and to which intermediary organizations (such as local authorities) or agencies (such as an insurance agency) the funds are allocated. Financing includes descript of which population groups have funded insurance coverage and what the level of coverage is (e.g., the health benefits package). Finally, financing takes account of how healthcare providers are remunerated.

The sources of financing in different countries vary. Funding may come from public or private sources. Public sources include taxes (general taxes or health-specific taxes) or public insurance (e.g., social insurance or publicly funded health insurance). Private sources of financing include private health insurance (through a combination of employer and personal contributions to the insurance premium), such as out-of-pocket expenditures, retail purchasing of care (such as dental services or drugs in some countries), or private payment for top–up insurance (in countries where the financing is predominantly from taxes [e.g., the United Kingdom] or statutory health insurance [e.g., France]), which could be individual or group insurance).

Insurance allows risks to be pooled; pooling enables people with varied levels of health needs to share their risk. Larger public insurance schemes (e.g., statutory health insurance) typically provide greater solidarity because such schemes draw contributions from all members of the population, regardless of ability to pay for insurance, bringing together higher- and lower-income groups as well as those who are healthy and those who may have multiple illnesses. Hence, higher-income citizens in countries with progressive tax schemes and those who are healthy subsidize those with lower incomes, illness, or high health risks.

The mix of financing sources vary from country to country as well (Table 2.6). Some countries' health systems are funded predominantly from general taxes, such as Canada and the United Kingdom, while others such as France or Germany predominantly from employers and employees through compulsory social insurance. Some are funded through compulsory private insurance, such as in Switzerland or the Netherlands, and others through voluntary private insurance, such as in the United States. However, almost all systems in the world have a mixture of funding from tax, social insurance, private insurance, and out-of-pocket payments. Each system has varying levels of contribution from each financing source, although rare exceptions such as Cuba (where currently there are no private insurance or private payments) exist.

The ways healthcare providers are paid also vary. Provider payment methods typically include

1. *Budget transfers*, where funds are transferred prospectively to providers to provide an agreed set of services for a given population.
2. *Salaries*, which could be fixed or performance related, based on the payment of a portion of funds following the achievement of pre-agreed results.
3. *Capitation payment*, which involves a fixed remuneration to healthcare providers for each person for whom they provide care. This could be simple capitation payment, which pays the same for each person, or a

Table 2.6 HEALTH SYSTEM FINANCING—DIFFERENT APPROACHES
ADOPTED BY COUNTRIES

	Tax	Statutory Health insurance		Voluntary Private Health Insurance (S = Supplementary)	Out-of-Pocket Payments
		Public	Private		
Brazil	☑			☑ S	☑
Canada	☑				☑
France		☑		☑ S	☑
Germany		☑	☑		☑
The Netherlands			☑		☑
Sweden	☑				☑
Switzerland	☑		☑	☑ S	☑
United Kingdom	☑			☑ S	☑
United States	☑			☑	☑

weighted (risk-adjusted) capitation payment with different weights attached to individual's characteristics (such as age, sex, socioeconomic status, location, and severity of illness).

4. *Fee-for-service*, which involves paying providers for each service they provide, either according to a preset and agreed fee schedule or following the submission of an invoice by providers setting the fee levels.

5. *Case-based payments*, which involve paying providers for a bundle of services they provide for an episode of care involving a procedure (e.g., hip operation or heart surgery) or an illness event (e.g., managing a person with a heart attack). The bundle of services for each case are typically predefined as is the remuneration. Examples of case-based systems include diagnosis-related groups, bundled payment, or its many variants across the world.

Payment mechanisms influence the behavior of healthcare providers by creating different kinds of incentives. In most countries, governments and payers use a mix of provider reimbursement systems to achieve health system objectives and goals (Table 2.7).

Table 2.7 PROVIDER PAYMENT MECHANISMS, INCENTIVES, AND PROVIDER BEHAVIOR

Provider Payment Mechanism	Cost per Unit	Service per Case	Volume of Services	Risk Selection
Global budget	– –	– –	–	0
Fee-for-service	– –	+ +	+ +	0
Capitation	– –	– –	– –	+ +
Case-based	– –	– –	+ +	+

Abbreviations: – –, strong incentive to reduce; –, moderate incentive to reduce; 0, no clear incentive' + moderate incentive to increase; ++, strong incentive to increase.

Key Questions

1. Where do the funds to support statutory health insurance come from?
2. What can you learn about priorities for health by comparing the level of funding with other national expenditure areas?
3. How are the funds allocated—young–old, rich–poor, urban–rural?
4. What does this allocation pattern tell you about the country's objectives regarding health?
5. What pattern do you see in the use of provider payment methods to influence healthcare provider behavior?

Group Task

What provider payment method might you use to expand utilization of a new service, improve the effectiveness of healthcare services (services that are high quality and beneficial to users), or improve efficiency or productivity. Record your responses in the Table 2.8.

Table 2.8 GROUP TASK ON PROVIDER PAYMENT MECHANISMS

	Expand Utilization	Improve Effectiveness	Improve Efficiency
Provider Payment Method			

Resource management is the process by which nations generate and distribute physical, technological (e.g., health technologies [medicines, diagnostics] and/or technologies for health [technologies developed in other sectors, such as computing, communication, supply chain management, but applied to health), and human and intellectual resources. An important component of this process is how these resources are allocated and made available to different parts of the health system, such as different geographies and populations.

One of the most important functions of a government is the process by which it decides how to invest and distribute its resources. These functions deeply influence the design and performance of health systems, what kind of care is available, and from whom, where, and when. Countries vary in the process and criteria they use in allocating their resources. Methods range from rational assessment of need and use of economic evaluation methods, such as cost-effectiveness analysis to determine which polices and interventions should be funded, to ethical considerations that take into equity, and methods that consider industrial and political and citizen influence. Most, however, share a similar process pathway; they relegate this activity largely to politicians and government. Budgets, specifically their creation and use, are a feature of every country's approach to shaping development priorities, in healthcare as in all government domains.

Your job is to determine and describe how your country sets its funding priorities for healthcare. You should examine your country, looking for good and bad ways it allocates resources. Harmful processes include those that are secret processes for decision-making; hidden decisions; have special political interests; are inequitable; provider-, payer-, or industry-influenced; or driven by self-interested demands of special disease groups or by unaffordable expectations. These processes can all be seen as suboptimal but are unfortunately real ways that priorities can be set. Those processes that are transparent, fair, just, socially responsive, and insulated from special interests are desirable. Some countries have evidence-based priority-setting, which is sheltered from special influences and committed to rational decision-making informing budgets and benefits. We expect you to have a good idea of how decisions in your country are made and what you see as its strengths and weaknesses with regard to using money wisely and for the best health results.

We follow with some examples of best practices of priority-setting to help you diagnose how your study country makes allocational decisions.

How are decisions made to determine how resources are used to provide services? Good priority-setting involves various stakeholders with different perspectives, including politicians, policymakers, managers, experts, patient groups, caretakers, members of civil society, the broader electorate, and, in low- and middle-income countries that receive overseas development assistance, the donor countries and/or agencies that provide financial and technical assistance.

Priority setting and resource allocation involves making choices. In your review, you should assess the following important considerations, namely:

1. Who decides?
2. How is the priority setting process structured ?
3. Is the process transparent?
4. On what basis are decisions made?
5. Who ultimately receives the benefits?
6. Is the process consistent with the values and attitudes of the citizens of the country?

Defining a clear, inclusive, and transparent deliberative process for priority-setting is critically important because citizens and decision makers have different ethical positions on priorities and fairness. There are competing demands on resources, and decisions often lead to winners and losers.

Accountability for reasonableness is one approach that enables the development of clear and inclusive priority-setting and management of resources. The accountability for reasonableness framework emphasizes procedural justice to achieve a clear, inclusive, and repeatable deliberative process, with public record.[17] The approach embodies four principles that guide the priority-setting process, namely:

1. Publicity (transparency, including reasons for the priority-setting process).
2. Relevant reasons (as judged by appropriate stakeholders).
3. Revisability (in light of new evidence, arguments, appeals).
4. Enforceability (assurance that other conditions are met).[17]

The principles embodied in the accountability for reasonableness framework have been applied flexibly in different settings and levels (e.g., Canada, Mexico, Norway, Sweden, and the United Kingdom). Collectively, the normative, contextual, technical, and institutional considerations influence what is prioritized, where resources are allocated, and who benefits.

Once a priority-setting process is agreed upon, or once resource allocation decisions must be made, the policymakers need to decide where the resources are allocated and on what basis. Countries typically use multiple criteria when deciding where to allocate resources. These include (Figure 2.3)

1. Normative considerations relating to values of the citizens (what they want their policymakers to do by exercising their rights in elections to vote for politicians or political parties) and values of policymakers;
2. Contextual considerations—for example, the level of need (the burden of disease and its distribution);
3. Institutional considerations, namely the resources and capabilities available in the health system, and the institutional setting in a country (such as laws and regulations; e.g., the laws in some countries or constitutions define health as a right, enabling citizens to challenge governments in courts to have access to new medicines or technologies).
4. Technical considerations, such as economic evaluation of interventions and programs to ascertain their cost and effectiveness (Figure 2.3).

Normative considerations are important when setting priorities. Here the prevailing values of the government, minister, and the electorate influence what is prioritized. For example, an electorate or government with *liberal*

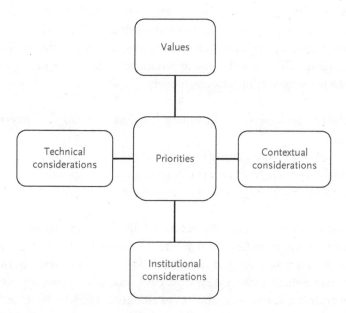

Figure 2.3 Priority setting: key considerations.

values might emphasize rights of individuals to choose and pay for health, encouraging individual choice on interventions like insurance. In contrast, a government with *utilitarian* values might prioritize interventions that generate the greatest health for the greatest number of people—for example, the most cost-effective public health interventions, such as immunization, nutrition in children, sanitation, and hygiene. Conversely, a government with *communitarian* values might emphasize equity over cost-effectiveness by investing in interventions for conditions that disproportionately affect the poor or cause impoverishment.

Contextual considerations relate to the current and future burden of disease that needs addressing. For example, high infant and maternal mortality might call for programmatic investment in intensive prenatal outreach programs.

Technical considerations relate to economic valuation of the interventions that are considered for prioritization to ascertain which are cost-effective. These considerations reflect an orientation to those interventions whose high benefits and/or low costs put them at higher priority for investment.

Institutional considerations relate to existing laws, regulations, resources, and capabilities in the government or country that might enable or hinder introduction or scale up of those interventions that are prioritized—for example, investing in polyclinics if access is low because of inaccessibility.

These criteria are considered when decisions are made to allocate resources at various levels. For example, governments decide what proportion of country's wealth or government budget is allocated to health. Decisions also consider to which geographies or population groups the resources should be allocated and in what proportion. A further resource allocation decision involves to which domains of the health system the resources should be allocated (e.g., primary healthcare, hospitals, community-based services, or public health) and to which areas (e.g., infectious diseases, mental illness, cancer, lung disease, child health, women's health, palliative care, etc.).

A further resource allocation decision is made regarding the interventions, programs, medicines, or health technologies that should be funded. For example, planners must decide which interventions should be included in a benefits package, which population or patient groups receive these interventions, and to what extent. For example, should all individuals have access to a set of core set of services and interventions (as is the case in Canada, France, the United Kingdom, New Zealand, the Nordic countries in Europe, and others), or should the benefits packages vary as is the case in many Latin American countries and the United States? Furthermore, an important resource allocation question relates to the level of expensive but useful resources that should be allocated to individual patients—an especially challenging question as some interventions are very costly, and in the context of finite resources or budgets, each decision has an impact on the ability of the system to fund other interventions.

Priority-setting and resource allocation in some countries involves the combined use of economic and ethical methods to inform decisions. Economic methods strive toward allocative efficiency and ethical approaches toward fairness and justice.

The most commonly used economic evaluation method in priority setting is cost-effectiveness analysis, which considers the effect of an intervention in the context of its costs. Those interventions that meet a specified cost-effectiveness threshold in terms of the effect they produce on one's life (measured as quality-adjusted life years) for a given cost are recommended for use in public healthcare systems. Economic evaluations are used in different countries in health technology assessment to inform policies regarding new technologies, medicines, and healthcare services and to set priorities (Table 2.9).

Effective priority-setting is essential in deciding on a health system design. Careful priority-setting leads to efficient allocation of resources, which can help achieve improved health, economic, and political outcomes. Conversely, misallocation of resources can have negative consequences for health outcomes, can adversely affect economic outcomes, and may have undesirable political outcomes as poor health and economic outcomes lead to unsatisfied electorate. However, not all countries use economic evaluation for priority-setting, and even those that do typically consider multiple criteria when setting priorities. Priorities should be set so as to achieve *value-for-money*, by allocating resources to effective interventions and delivering them in an efficient way, while also ensuring equity and responsiveness to realize *value-for-many*.

This framework falls in line with recent research and publications aimed at guiding thinking on prioritization. For example, the WHO Consultative Group on Equity and Universal Health Coverage recommends that when setting priorities in relation to universal health coverage, countries should consider

1. *Categorizing services into priority classes*—use cost-effectiveness, priority to the worse off, and financial risk protection as criteria.
2. *Expanding priority services*—expand coverage of high-priority services to everyone and eliminate out-of-pocket payments, while increasing mandatory, progressive prepayment with pooling of funds.
3. *Including more people* in universal health coverage—ensure disadvantaged groups are not left behind.

Table 2.9 HEALTH TECHNOLOGY ASSESSMENT AND HOW IT IS USED
IN DIFFERENT COUNTRIES

	Agency	Application	Purpose
Australia	Medical Services Advisory Committee (MSAC) and Pharmaceutical Benefits Advisor Committee (PBAC)	MSAC: New service PBAC: New pharmaceuticals	Funding decisions regarding health technologies
Canada	Canadian Agency for Drugs and Technologies in Health		
Germany	Institute for Quality and Efficiency in Health Care	Pharmaceuticals	To ascertain an upper limit for reimbursement of pharmaceuticals
United Kingdom	National Institute for Health and Clinical Excellence	Pharmaceuticals, medical devices, diagnostic techniques, surgical procedures, other therapeutic technologies, health promotion activities	To appraise clinical and cost-effectiveness of interventions and recommend for use (or decline) in the national health system

When allocating resources an important consideration is management and accountability. The best designed systems have processes in place to monitor performance, detect errors or fraud, measure results, and determine effectiveness and efficiency of resource allocation decisions.

Health System Outputs

Health system outputs are the services delivered to the citizens, including

1. Public health services, such as health education, promotion, and preventive services, and
2. Personal healthcare services, such as diagnosis, treatment, care, and palliation provided in patients' home, in the community, in primary healthcare settings, and in hospitals.

Public Health Services

Public health services relate to broad range of services related to health promotion, health protection, and disease prevention. Health promotion services are designed to promote population health and well-being by addressing inequalities and the broader social and environmental determinants of health and empowering individuals and populations to have healthier lifestyles and behaviors across life course.

- Health protection services are designed to protect individuals and populations from communicable diseases and environmental risks and hazards.
- Disease prevention involves services provided mainly by health professionals at primary, secondary, and tertiary levels. Examples of primary prevention include routine immunization programs, environmental interventions aimed at reducing accidents (seat belts in cars and safe environments for children), healthy eating, and exercise. Examples of secondary prevention include routine screening for diseases such as major forms of cancer for early diagnosis and treatment and provision of treatment to maintain health or slowdown disease progression (e.g., antihypertensive medication or the use of lipid lowering agents). Tertiary prevention is aimed at improving quality of life by reducing disability, limiting or delaying complications of disease, and restoring function. This is done by treating the disease and providing rehabilitation—for example, rehabilitation following cerebrovascular stroke.
- Health promotion, health protection, and disease prevention services are informed by contextually relevant intelligence derived from (i) effective surveillance of population health and well-being, including surveillance of health risks, determinants of health, and incidence of prevalence of diseases; (ii) monitoring and response to health hazards and emergencies; and (iii) ongoing needs assessments to ascertain current and future health needs.
- Population analytics are helping public health. Advances in digital data, creation of large data sets, computing, and analytical techniques have enabled better stratification of population groups to develop *precision health* services to better target services and engage individuals to mitigate health risk and to maintain and improve health.

Personal Healthcare Services

Personal healthcare services are those delivered to individual patients. Medical care is the primary personal healthcare service. It is provided in many different settings, such as home, in the community, in primary healthcare delivery settings, and in hospitals. Personal healthcare services are delivered by many different medical providers, including doctors, nurses, pharmacists, and technicians, all with a single patient as the target.

Personal healthcare services dominate the healthcare scene but are not without substantial controversies and problems. There are several important considerations in relation to personal healthcare services in health systems. For example, there are differences of opinion and considerable variation in practices regarding comprehensiveness of the services that are offered; the balance between hospital services and those provided in primary healthcare and in the community; continuity of care, namely the coordination of patients' journey in health systems along the care continuum through effective referral and counterreferral; methods of reimbursement and incentives; and doubt and debate about the proper mix of individual services to meet current and future needs.

A further consideration relates to the mix of publicly and privately provided health services and the ability of the health system to use the available assets in the country to achieve desired health system outcomes.

Health System Objectives

Every health system produces a balance of objectives (Figure 2.4). The equilibrium is informed by the values of citizens, the values of policymakers, and other factors that inform resource allocation decisions.

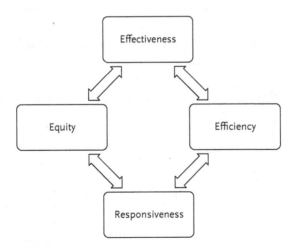

Figure 2.4 Achieving a balanced output of health services in health systems.

To achieve desired outcomes, a health system should provide services (outputs) that are effective, efficient, equitable, and responsive. *Effectiveness* refers to provision of the *right services* (those that are beneficial to users). *Efficiency* refers to provision of health services in the *right way*, so that scarce resources are appropriately used. *Equity* means providing access to services to citizens in a fair way so that they reach the *right people*. *Responsiveness* means the services provided are *relevant* to the needs of citizens and person-centered. The latter refers to satisfying the preferences of individuals and communities and empowering them.

Effectiveness relates to the extent to which a desired outcome is achieved when a cost-effective intervention is applied to a population. It includes an assessment of technical quality of clinical care and the extent to which evidence-based interventions are used.

Efficiency is the capacity of a system to produce the maximum goods and services for a given amount of resource. Efficiency refers to (i) macro-economic efficiency—the level of health expenditure as a fraction of the gross domestic product—and (ii) microeconomic efficiency—namely *allocative efficiency* (producing the right outputs to achieve goals; i.e., *what mix of services are produced* using available resources to maximize a combination of health outcomes and user satisfaction) and *technical efficiency* (producing outputs at minimum costs; i.e. *how the services are produced*—inputs or costs should be minimized for target output).

Equity relates to fairness in the allocation of resources or services among different individuals or groups. It also encompasses access to health services by population segments and their subsequent health outcomes. It considers equality of health service coverage and differing ability of various groups to access care and treatment, and how those with higher needs receive resources and services commensurate with those needs. Finally, equity refers to whether those in equal need are treated equally, irrespective of other characteristics such as ability to pay.

Responsiveness relates to the ability of the health system to meet legitimate expectations of citizens in relation to perceived service accessibility, quality, and experience as patients.

Group Exercise

Work in your groups to identify two recent policies in a country you are familiar with aimed at improving health system objectives. Explain what prompted the policymakers to introduce these policies. Document your answers in Table 2.10.

Table 2.10 COUNTRY EXAMPLES OF POLICIES TO IMPROVE HEALTH
SYSTEMS OBJECTIVES

	Effectiveness	Efficiency	Equity	Responsiveness
Policy 1				
Policy 2				

Health System Outcomes

Health system outcomes are the results that a system produces. These relate to population health, financial protection, and user satisfaction (Box 2.3). The goal of health systems should be to improve both the level and the distribution of these outcomes, so that the system benefits everyone equitably.

Box 2.3: HEALTH SYSTEM OUTCOMES

Population health is concerned with both the level and distribution of health (e.g., as measured by life expectancy at birth or at age 30 or 60 years), mortality (mortality levels), or burden of disease (as measured by disability-adjusted life years), as well as specific population health outcomes of interest—such as infant or under-five mortality rate, maternal mortality ratio, standardized mortality rate for key diseases, or premature mortality from key diseases. Population health is measured by indicators such as average life expectancy at birth or death rates for various conditions (e.g., for pneumonia, HIV, malaria, or tuberculosis) or population groups (e.g., infant mortality rate, under-five mortality rate, maternal mortality ratio).

Financial protection relates to fairness in health financing (distribution of health expenditures) and the extent of financial risk protection for general population and specific population segments, as measured by levels of out-of-pocket expenditures as a percentage of total health spending and impoverishing health expenditures incurred by individuals in different income groups). Out-of-pocket expenditures deter individuals from accessing health services, while impoverishing health expenditures push individuals affected by an illness and their families into poverty, with further adverse health consequences.

User satisfaction assesses its citizens' satisfaction with their health system, which is an end in itself but also effects health outcomes because low satisfaction levels adversely influence user engagement and use of health services.

Table 2.11 COUNTRY EXAMPLES OF POLICIES TO IMPROVE HEALTH SYSTEMS OUTCOMES

	Health Outcomes	Financial Protection	User Satisfaction
Policy 1			
Policy 2			
Policy 3			

Group Exercise: Policies to Improve Health System Outcomes

Work in your groups to identify a recent policy by in a country you are familiar with aimed at improving health system outcomes. Explain what prompted the policymakers to introduce this policy. Document your answers in the Table 2.11.

NOTE

* A note to the course director: If possible, organize student choices so that two or more groups choose the same country. Cross-group comparisons facilitate learning.

CHAPTER 3

How Did We Get Here?

Historical Megatrends in Health and Medical Care

Those who cannot remember the past are condemned to repeat it.
—Attributed to George Santayana

The perspective of this chapter is historical. We present a brief overview of modern healthcare. We trace its development and the post–Second World War (WWII) trends that led to our present-day approach to health system design in middle- and high-income countries. We summarize the major trends in benefits, costs, public attitudes and beliefs, and consumer responses to medical care. We reflect on what forces have brought us to our current successes and raise upcoming challenges in improving health and healthcare.

THE EVOLUTION OF HEALTH SYSTEMS

Each country has its own health system with a unique and distinctive profile, and the dissimilarities among national systems initially appear great. Nations differ in what they consider good health, how much they allocate to achieve it, and in how they set priorities among healthcare services. Nations strike their own balances between medical care and public health, publicly versus privately financed services, universal versus selective medical insurance and access, primary care versus hospital-based delivery, publicly owned and operated versus private management of resources, and so forth.

Our contention, however, is that all national health systems operate aligned with some surprisingly common historical trends, features, and constraints, even though each country may operationalize its system in different ways. We call these commonalities "megatrends," with the starting point of the trend commencing shortly after WWII when most of the modern features of health systems in high-income countries began to accelerate. An understanding of these megatrends makes it possible not only to assess how individual countries have adapted, but also to discern how and if these trends will influence the effectiveness of any proposed future changes.

A DEVELOPMENTAL FRAMEWORK

In the following section, we will describe the historical trends of the health of populations today and the developmental breakthroughs that have gotten us to our current state. We organize this historical overview using a framework consisting of four essential parameters of a successful health system (Figure 3.1). These are (i) effectiveness, which correlates with quality; (ii) equity, or the degree to which the health system is solidly behind extending accessible and affordable healthcare services to all citizens;

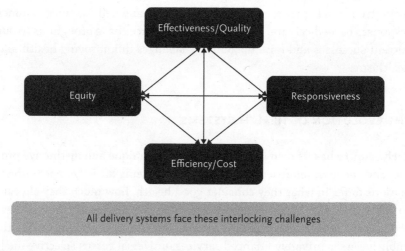

Figure 3.1 Essential parameters for health system success.

(iii) responsiveness, which is the capacity of a health system to deliver a product that satisfies patient-centered demand and personal expectations; and (iv) efficiency, which reflects cost.

These four parameters comprise the value-for-money of a health system. The system produces health, social solidarity, and consumer satisfaction at a cost to the nation. These three benefits divided by cost equals the value produced.

Using this framework, we present our view of the long-term trends of health systems. Our data and insights are drawn from publications from the Organization for Economic Cooperation and Development (OECD),[1] the World Health Organization (WHO)[2] Commonwealth Fund,[3] and the World Bank.[4] The OECD countries are 37 industrialized countries that represent almost two-thirds of global gross domestic product (GDP); the organization produces health-related and other reports. We will discuss each megatrend and then, in the next chapter, drill down on healthcare delivery models adopted in individual countries.

THE HISTORICAL PERFORMANCE OF HEALTHCARE

Quality/Effectiveness of Medical Care in Middle- and High-Income Countries

Trend 1: Gains in the Health Status of Nations

A generally accepted high-level measure of health systems performance (as well as medical care quality and of public health interventions and trends in social determinants of health) is overall health status. Population health in middle- and high-income countries has improved remarkably since WWII. Longevity has increased dramatically in all OECD countries. Life expectancy in them was 48.2 years immediately after WWII and has risen to an average of just over 80 today. Other measures of health outcomes have also improved markedly, such as quality-adjusted life years (QALYs), avoidable mortality or morbidity, disability-adjusted life years, and other measures such as health-adjusted life years.

Specific post-WWII threats to health have diminished. Maternal and infant mortality have declined markedly. Maternal deaths in high-income countries have become relatively rare. Across all OECD countries, infant mortality in the first year has dropped from 30 to about 4 deaths per 1,000 live births. Premature mortality (avoidable early deaths) has decreased by over 50% since 1970. Although Covid-19 has exposed some overconfidence and complacency, the risks of epidemics have been decreasing. For example, in addition to smallpox, polio has been virtually eradicated globally, and new epidemics—such as AIDS—have mostly been under control with numbers of new infections and deaths on the decline. Vaccines have greatly reduced the impact of measles and influenza while the illnesses from other lower-morbidity viral epidemics like chicken pox have been mitigated. Advances in diagnosis and treatment have improved predicted disability and death from many cancers, coronary heart disease, infections, and strokes. Food safety has greatly reduced the risk of food-borne diseases in First World countries.

Medical care and public health have each contributed significantly to the overall improved health status of populations in middle- and high-income countries. Of course, we know that a number of factors other than medical care and public health have contributed to improved population health, even as some new ones threaten to undermine our gains in health. Even accounting for the absence of major wars and the growing wealth of nations, the public credits healthcare as a major intervention in achieving the good results we have enjoyed.

Trend 2: The Successes of Scientific Discovery

Scientific discovery and engineering advances have transformed what medical care can offer, bringing us much of our current medical success while also presenting us with upcoming challenges. Although hard to believe today, the only genetics known at the onset of WWII was rudimentary Mendelian inheritance. DNA and its role had not yet been discovered. X-rays were our sole imaging technology. There were no functional computers until the ENIAC (the Electrical Numerical Integrator and Computer) became operational in 1946. Surgeons could only operate with open exposure of their target and had no means to correct physical abnormalities in the heart. At the beginning of WWII, sulfa had just come into use and was the only antibiotic. We had no ability to culture cells *in vitro* and study their functions.

The scientific basis of biology has strengthened immeasurably with the discovery of DNA and genetic interventions, advanced engineering, and the digital revolution. To the authors, whose careers started several decades or so after the end of the WWII, the advances are dramatic and amazing in scope. These scientific developments have supported improvements in diagnosis and treatment, stemming especially from breakthroughs in antibiotics, interventional cardiology, cancer treatments, smoking cessation initiatives, improved preventive care, and increasing sophistication in the organization and financing of medical care to make it more accessible and effective.

Advances have transformed what we know and can do. Drugs now deliver treatment modalities not even imagined 50 years ago—utilizing macromolecules, antibodies, and genetic manipulations, for example. Thanks to our knowledge of how the genome works, we now have a growing understanding of disease and an expanding array of interventions that capitalize on our ability to actually manipulate the working mechanisms of our defenses and vulnerabilities. Detailed genetic information from individuals and their diseases is enabling personalized targeting of interventions to improve results in, for example, cancer treatment. Several vaccines protecting against Covid-19 depend on sophisticated genetic manipulation. Advances in engineering and computing have given us microsurgery with keyhole instruments, amazing imaging such as MRI (magnetic resonance imaging), and manipulations through catheters that can even replace heart valves percutaneously, bringing us closer to same-day valve replacement. Surgical and other interventions are safer and more effective, and recovery is faster.

The scientific advances in public health have also been notable. Improvements in knowledge and effectiveness of interventions in areas such as epidemiology, social marketing, environmental safety, vaccination, smoking regulation, nutritional habits, and health education have proven how cost-effective public health can be.

Trend 3: Effectiveness of Medical Care

The effectiveness of medical care has steadily improved. Effectiveness research has expanded. Epidemiology has provided research methods that help us understand patterns of disease and information about which interventions do and do not work. With advanced study design and methods such as randomized controlled trials, we have evolved a solid methodology to vet new medical interventions and conduct surveillance.

Research, training methods, sources of continuing education, and communication about best medical practices are now globally similar. More is known about what constitutes appropriate care and why. Medical processes have improved and standardized, thus leading to a generally high understanding of what is appropriate to provide. Process criteria may differ slightly from country to country, but they all stem from the same research and literature base. The variation among nations is relatively small. Practitioners, teachers, and even patients can expect a common approach to the medical management of health and sickness regardless of the country they are in, despite variation in the organization and financing of the delivery of care.

Trend 4: Improvements in Healthcare Services Delivery

As science, technology, and education have increased the scope of healthcare, so have nations progressively improved their capacity to deliver care. The medical workforce has become more sophisticated and grown to meet demand. Healthcare management, measurement and accountability, distribution, and financing have expanded the accessibility of populations to healthcare services.

Almost all experts believe that first contact, accessible primary care is essential for a well-functioning health system. A 1978 landmark international conference in Alma Ata first designated primary care as the *sine qua non* of healthcare delivery. The WHO, countries, and other organizations have cited the importance of primary care, and it is universally recognized as the foundation of health systems. Over the past half century, primary care services based on allopathic doctors and advanced practice nurses have grown and augmented services formerly provided by community health workers, barefoot doctors (China), and Feldshers (Russia).

Primary care has greatly improved first access to medical care in most countries. Primary care now delivers medically sophisticated first-contact, generalist care. Primary care capacity and capability have upgraded tremendously. Education systems are producing the kinds of doctors and other health personnel that are most needed and that fill workforce specialty deficiencies. Training of doctors has improved.

Hospitals have become increasingly specialized centers of medical delivery. Specialists are generally higher paid and more highly regarded by the public. The costs of secondary or tertiary care by specialists and hospitals have grown disproportionately, and these expenses are generally the largest single item in most middle and higher-income countries' medical care budgets. Nevertheless, their cost has been mitigated by a real trend toward increased efficiency. New research has safely nudged hospital stays shorter. Much hospitalization has shifted to day surgery with the advent of keyhole and other technologies shortening length of stays.

Citizens have become more informed patients. Health literacy has improved through education and the prominence of health issues in the media. Some cultural barriers to effective care have been recognized and reduced.

Good management practices have infiltrated healthcare in the past half century. Medical care's growth has increased the need for better management. Medical care has specialized tremendously, delivery has become more fragmented, the product is more complicated, and the need for integration has grown. There is simply much greater process complexity and throughput, as well as complicated payment and reimbursement systems, demanding efficiency, effectiveness, and service. In addition, as medical care has come to consume more of the productive capacity of nations, payers are under growing pressure to deliver more value for money, and even to halt the rise of medical service spending. In response, governments, insurers, provider organizations, and even small practices have incorporated best business practices in leadership, delivery design, human resources, standardization, training, accounting, and measurement and accountability.

Management methods have become increasing sophisticated over time. W. Edwards Deming, a groundbreaking engineer who transformed Japanese manufacturing, established the use of statistical process control as a method of continuous improvement. It quickly spread to medical care and has led to a worldwide quality improvement movement. Formal quantitative descriptive methods were the foundation of modern systems thinking through the work of Jay Forrester at Massachusetts Institute of Technology.

Further, as medical care has expanded, the structure and methods of its delivery workforce have shifted. The days of medical care as a sole-proprietor cottage industry are fading rapidly. Primary care clinicians are more likely now to practice in groups and in multiprofessional teams. In the United States, and beginning elsewhere, primary care groups are being incorporated into vertically integrated organizations with hospitals at their center. Specialists are dependent on and aggregated in hospitals.

Reimbursement methods are becoming more sophisticated. Fee-for-service reimbursement is only one of many ways that clinicians are now compensated—many are salaried or regularly receive payments detached from services delivered and rather pegged to their number of patients (known as capitation). Many reimbursement and financing mechanisms have been designed to rein in rising costs.

In every sector of healthcare, measurement of inputs and outcomes is recognized now as essential in decision-making and prediction. It is a truism that "without measurement, there is no management." Without such measurement, market forces don't work since neither buyer nor seller is able to know the value of what they are bargaining about or estimate risks and benefits. Whether in research, individual patient care interventions, or managing an organization, measuring and assessing the results against those that are expected and using the data to analyze, understand, assess, predict, and adjust the next intervention have become common and expected practices.

The use of research evidence to determine what benefits should be covered in national healthcare programs has become well-established. A variety of tools, measurement scales, and processes to assess cost–benefit are available now. In association with the development and application of these quantitative methodologies, some governments have realized the need to make their own decisions about the cost, effectiveness, and benefits of new diagnostic methods and treatments. Organizations have emerged, usually quasi-independent non-governmental in form, to gather evidence and present cost-effectiveness and benefit coverage recommendations to guide what would be covered in population-based systems of health care. The best example of this is NICE (the National Institute for Health and Care Excellence) in England. Since its start in 1999, NICE has been an independent body responsible for developing information, standards, and guidance about the cost-effectiveness of interventions on health and social care system. Its evidence-based, expert-assisted recommendations are the basis by which the National Health Service (NHS) determines which services to cover and what process standards in care are the gold standard.

Emerging Threats to Medical Care Benefits

Health systems in middle- and high-income countries are running into head winds. The foremost threat is rising costs, which we discuss later in this section. In addition, however, there is a range of other problems that are creating challenges for health systems. These are summarized in Box 3.1.

Box 3.1: THREATS TO THE BENEFITS FROM HEALTHCARE

- As medical care has grown, a ceiling effect is emerging that limits the level of health improvement that can be generated through individual care and lowers the cost-effectiveness of each additional gain.
- The emergence of new life-style diseases and complications, inadequately managed by the current medical model.

- Keeping people alive longer is creating a burden of disability.
- Public health is growing more vital to improving health than medical care but has fallen far behind individual care in its proportion of national investment in healthcare in almost all countries.
- Primary care is struggling to attract, motivate, and retain doctors. Specialism is growing ever more popular.
- Corporatization of healthcare is growing in both public and private medical delivery. As business takes over many healthcare functions, it can be seen as an opportunity for improvement in management or as a threat to the autonomy, motivation, and accountability of doctors—or both.
- Upgraded management is lagging as a force for improvement in benefits; gains in efficiency and effectiveness have only led to trivial gains in improving healthcare and health.
- The big breakthroughs in digital infrastructure that have transformed other industries have been slow to make a difference in medical care.
- Little of the available research and development funding in medical care has gone to what some have called *delivery science*—the analysis, design, and testing of new structural systems aimed at getting the right medical services out to the right people at the right time at the right price.

Equity and Accessibility to Medical Care

Trend 1: The Goal of Health for All as a Right and the Means to Achieve It

Almost all high-income countries have endorsed their citizens' right to healthcare services, and the WHO emphasized that health is a fundamental human right in its 1948 founding charter. The charter states that "the enjoyment of the highest attainable standard of health is one of the fundamental rights of every human being without distinction of race, religion, and political belief, economic or social condition."[5] To operationalize that goal, medical services must be accessible and affordable.

Much progress has been made in achieving the WHO's 1948 goal. Of major importance to increasing the availability of clinical services and improving health is the way nations design and deliver insurance and medical care. Medical services have become progressively more accessible, acceptable, and equitable in most countries over the past 70 or more years.

Health insurance is available to all citizens in almost all middle- or high-income countries, and financial barriers to use have declined in all countries save the United States, which is the prime example of a system that is still unaffordable for many. The United States has been unable to provide universal health insurance. Many middle- and lower-income citizens face barriers to accessing care. Moreover, the trend in the United States is for rising costs to be passed on to patients, so financial barriers to use are rising.

Since WWII, much progress has been made in organizational support to improve health status. The WHO, a United Nations agency, articulated ambitious goals in the preamble to its founding constitution adopted in 1946 (entered into force in 1948) in which it defined health as "a state of complete physical, mental and social well-being and not merely the absence of disease or infirmity."[5] Over the years, the WHO has supported groundbreaking conferences, such as the Alma Ata Conference in 1978, which declared the centrality of primary care to achieve "health for all," and in its Global Strategy published in 1981, which challenged the world to achieve "health for all by the year 2000."

Improvement of health equity has emerged as a clear priority for global institutions and United Nations member states. Healthcare for all citizens is a widely accepted goal. Few would argue today that nations, businesses, or other organizations are not obligated to provide the means for their constituents to enjoy good health. Indeed, most countries have endorsed their responsibility for healthcare. The benefits—both individual and collective—from agreeing to that responsibility are clear.

Trend 2: Collective Insurance as the Means to Achieve Equal Access and Share Risk

Medical insurance has dramatically reduced the individual financial burden of accessing and using healthcare. A major barrier to medical services has always been that of individual financial risk and affordability. Who pays for medical care has shifted from individuals to pools of people that share the risk of costly care. Starting in the immediate postwar period, almost every country developed systems of insurance with collective resources to pay for access to needed medical care and protect individuals from unpredictable expenses associated with illness. In most OECD countries, financial barriers to use have mostly disappeared or been greatly reduced, and insurance has democratized access to healthcare services.

Universal health insurance as we know it today didn't gather steam until just after WWII. Precursors to this movement began in Germany in 1893 with Sickness Funds, supported first by employers. Although this type of pooled protection against loss of income during illness was adopted by many countries, in 1948 England was the first country to promise universal availability of healthcare that was "free at the point of use" and paid for by government through taxation. Since then, almost all developed countries and population groups except the United States have instituted national programs that reduce or eliminate the financial risk of medical care for all citizens.

The means by which nations provide universal health insurance varies greatly. Some, like England, build or contract healthcare services whose use is either free or close to it, while other countries mandate some mechanism for universal insurance coverage to pay for private services.

In most middle- and high-income countries, health insurance is heavily supported from collective sources. Countries have found a way to pay for these improvements in accessibility and clinical effectiveness. Healthcare has transitioned from households paying out of pocket to pooled financing. The sources of funding range from government to employer or employee, with some small, but decreasing, personal contributions at the time of use. The approaches for funding of health insurance vary from plans supported solely by government through taxation to others that require employers or individuals to pay a share of the collective insurance funds. No two countries or large businesses or organizations are identical in how this is done. Nevertheless, payers have usually stepped up to fund growing costs of medical care delivery. What varies is who pays, what services are covered, how much of the cost is borne by the individual user, and whether the health insurance function is government- or privately-run.

Trend 3: Recognition of the Importance of Providing Social Supports

The importance of allocating resources for social support rather than only to medical care is increasingly clear. But countries vary greatly in the degree to which their governments have come to support social care. European countries spend a higher proportion of their GDP on social support services than the United States. Scandinavian countries direct the most government resources to social support network activities. The results of these interventions on population health vary among countries, since many societal factors influence social and medical morbidity.

Quality of life has generally improved in middle- and high-income countries. Happiness, one measure of quality of life, is the result of complex interactions between health, well-being, and a multitude of other factors. However, the World Happiness Report 2020 concludes:

> The stronger social environment thereby leads to a significant reduction in the inequality of well-being (by about 13%). . . . Favorable social environments not

only raise the level of well-being but also improve its distribution. We conclude that social environments are of first-order importance for the quality of life.[6]

Happiness is higher in countries that exhibit social solidarity, trust in government, and social welfare investment.

Emerging Threats to Equity and Accessibility

Despite dramatic improvements in the health of nations, significant inequities and disparities persist. Health benefits are still unevenly distributed in middle- and high-income countries, especially among immigrant populations, racial and ethnic groups, other minorities, people from low socioeconomic backgrounds, and elderly people. Those with fewer educational opportunities consistently have poorer health outcomes than the general population. For these subpopulations, barriers to medical care are pervasive, and as a result—in combination with social determinants of health—improvements in health outcomes remain stagnant.

Increasing longevity creates a larger population of the elderly, frail, sick, poor, and dependent people who need help. Families are struggling to support aging seniors. Adequate resources are generally not available to provide comprehensive social supports for the elderly. Reduced government spending and services for social assistance have especially hurt the old and frail.

These circumstances are increasingly the health status challenges of the 21st century. Some countries recognize that social supports may reduce medical costs and therefore are relatively generous in the services they provide. Others primarily respond to the demand for medical care and offer little in the way of social support, either short or long term. As a consequence, some important health measures have lagged in low-income pockets of populations within countries whose overall status has improved. Perceived health status, for example, has barely budged in the past half century. As best as it can be measured, happiness has not widely increased in the new millennium. Social disruption, perhaps the greatest threat to happiness, has been on the rise globally and the consequences of Covid-19 on the economies of middle- and high-income countries portends a darkening rise of social distress.

Underuse of healthcare persists even with universal accessibility to care. While universal protection against financial risk has been a huge success in increasing access to medical services, other barriers have blocked availability. Among these are shortages in medical workforce (primary care doctors especially), geographic and transportation hurdles, cultural health beliefs, and education barriers.

Responsiveness and the Patient Experience

Trend 1: Little Change in the Patient Experience Unless You Can Pay for It

Healthcare has a disappointing record of responsiveness from its patients' point of view. Medical care has changed, if at all, for the worse over the past half century in its attention to the experience of patients. Delivery has evolved from a personal encounter with a general practitioner you knew, in a small, local office to a more technically oriented and bureaucratic encounter. Hospitals, growing ever more effective at producing specialized services, have remained forbidding experiences for patients. While medical care has become logistically available for more people over time, few citizens would applaud its responsiveness to its consumers. Medicine has fallen far behind other services, where the user experience and satisfaction are aggressively pursued.

Medical care remains a supplier- and product-driven industry. Doctors are primarily focused on producing good care and not on their patients' experience. The organization of healthcare delivery favors efficiency and satisfaction for the doctors and hospitals, rather than a pleasing experience for the patient.

Changing public expectations can erode perceptions of responsiveness, as well as affecting perceived equity and accessibility. There is a rising expectation of accessibility and service, accompanied by demanding behaviors and loss of positive regard for doctors over time. Regardless of the cause, self-interest, declining trust in professional expertise, and the idea that patients are consumers who need to be satisfied have combined to fuel higher expectations and demands from the public for access, treatments, and results. Declining respect for authority, expertise, and intellectual leadership in society at large has leaked into medical care, with more patients suspicious and skeptical. These factors inevitably strain the available service capacity and lead to overworked, stressed-out, and underappreciated caregivers.

Efficiency—The Costs of Medical Care

Trend 1: Progressive Increases in National Costs

The single largest expenditure in all middle- and high-income OECD countries is that of paying the costs of healthcare. The average expenditure is around 10% of their GDP. Of that amount, over 90% is spent on personal medical care. Individuals are mostly sheltered from these costs, but the annual rate of increase in national healthcare cost has on average outpaced GDP growth since WWII. Since 2000, middle- and high-income countries have experienced annual healthcare cost increases averaging between 3% and 4%, a rate which has consistently outpaced the annual growth of GDP.

Why have the costs of delivering medical care to a population steadily risen for more than half a century? Much of this can be attributed to increased quantity and effectiveness of today's available services and technologies, as previously noted. The causes of rising costs (summarized in Box 3.2) vary but reflect increased sophistication of medical care, aging of the population, multimorbidity, and the proliferation of new diagnostic and treatment modalities, coupled with demand from those with insurance to receive more—more hospital and office visits with doctors and nurses and more and newer tests and treatments. Even in the face of increased demand, there remain active debates about the degree to which improvements in longevity, morbidity, and other health indices are the result of improved care versus public health and socioeconomic changes.

Box 3.2: MAJOR CONTRIBUTORS TO INCREASING MEDICAL CARE EXPENDITURES IN HIGH-INCOME COUNTRIES

- Aging of populations—the gains in longevity create a growing proportion of elderly citizens who are sicker than the national average.
- Epidemiological transition—to lifestyle diseases and the growth of chronic illness occuring across the age spectrum.
- Rising citizens expectations coupled with protecting them from the direct costs of care.
- New technologies—continuous invention of new tests and treatments.
- Populist political pressures—increasing demand pressures governments to pay for more benefits.
- Absence of constraining forces—such as competition, financial barriers to care, and government regulatory limits to benefits.
- Healthcare as a citizen's right—extending subsidized medical care to all adds to direct costs.
- Professional and scientific dominance—decisions about allocation are influenced by the public's belief in the superior value of medical care over other priorities, including social determinants of illness.

Trend 2: How Nations Pay for Healthcare

Someone has to pay for healthcare delivery. Most do so through pooling the risk of illness and subsequent utilization of medical care through health insurance—that is, pooling healthy people with those at risk of illness and spreading the associated costs among the entire group. In some cases, like England, the government operates as a single payer, covering the costs of all citizens by funding healthcare delivery through general tax revenues and national insurance. In others, such as Germany and Switzerland, universal health insurance is mandated by defining the rules and enabling all insurers to compete to attract customers. In the diversity of models, sources of funding can vary from taxation, to employer-based payment, to individually purchased health insurance.

Emerging Threats from Unchecked Rises in Healthcare Costs

The greatest threat to universal, personally affordable, accessible medical care is cost itself. Rising costs are a built-in feature of current health system structure. We believe that contemporary healthcare insurance design is built on a structural model that stimulates costs to rise and guarantees that nations will inevitably be forced to respond. This argument is presented in detail later in this book. Without mitigating this systems flaw, rising costs will ultimately reduce needed services and possibly even price universal medical care out of reach again.

How fast the health system reaches its limits depends on how well it is managed. Improving its efficiency and effectiveness, setting limits, defining and prioritizing desired benefits, and agreeing expectations are examples of mitigating actions. Policy interventions to moderate costs have ranged from actions such as improving performance, to reserving individual medical care to those who need it and are likely to benefit the most, to rationing based upon ability to pay.

Systems Constraints that Limit National Funding of Health Services

As medical care has improved and the expectation of its use has risen, demand has steadily increased. Both doctors and patients have fueled this rise. First, medical care's array of new products and services is never-ending, doctors want to provide it, and patients want access to them. Supply drives demand.

Second, healthcare is financed in a way that stimulates demand. It represents one of system theory's classic archetypes called The Tragedy of the Commons, in which a scarce resource is systematically over-utilized when the collective benefit (e.g., health insurance) is subsidized and its cost to the user is less than the cost to produce it. It is named after a classic example in which herders destroyed grass-rich town Commons areas where grazing was free; as more and more took advantage, the resource was destroyed by unchecked overuse. When the costs of using medical care are subsidized, patients are less constrained by financial costs that modulate overuse. According to systems thinking, the growth of medical care expenditures is structurally pre-determined. Costs will progressively increase until countervailing balancing forces bring it to a limit. Sustainability of the shared resource will eventually become a priority.

Third, insurance pools are subject to moral hazard and adverse selection. That is, individuals will game the system in some way that favors them, driving up the costs of providing medical services. In medical care, moral hazard can range from jumping the queue to misrepresenting personal data that provides the individual access to scarce resource.

Sensible Initial Adjustments

There are effective actions that nations can take to delay hitting the limits of national expenditures on medical services. These initiatives seek to make the system run better. The undertakings improve outcomes while holding costs in check.

Increase Cost-effectiveness Improving the performance of a health system will increase value-for-money. Any enhancement of benefits more than their added costs, elimination of unnecessary or low-value activities, and improvements in appropriateness of decisions will stretch the limited resources available.

Manage Better Improvements in efficiency leading to reductions in waste, re-work, duplication, and work-arounds can improve value-for-money.

Agree on Expectations The level of citizen satisfaction with the health system's results determines the threshold of acceptable system performance. If expectations are defined, realistic, and agreed by citizens, satisfaction can be achieved at lower national investment.

Innovation Creative design and good management of the shared insurance resource can make it more efficient and effective and can increase benefits and lower cost increases for a time. The better the structural design and its management, the longer that nations can sustain insurance and satisfy public demand.

Desperate Measures

In the face of public demand for increases in services and relief from costs, governments or businesses may understandably give way to demand. In covering rising costs, they may reduce short term pressures but expose the health of the population to long-term threats, as follows.

Drain Resources from Other Priorities Medical care competes with other priorities that need to be considered as deserving of collective support. Leaders of nations, organizations, or businesses have many challenges. Goals should be set in the context of a strategy for national success. Government should allocate resources as needed to achieve the priorities among these goals. Access to healthcare can drain resources from other priorities such as public health, education, needed infrastructure, social welfare, defense, and retirement support.

An example of the damage caused by diverting resources to personal medical care is under-resourced public health. As medical care's proportion of national or business budgets has grown, public health has stagnated, and its share of GDP has declined. Public health, in most developed countries, has not come close to matching the investment in individual medical care even though investment in public health interventions usually yields far higher returns on the level of population health achieved for money spent. From the public policy point of view, this allocation of resources is suboptimal.

It is understandable why nations are tempted to divert resources from other priorities to fund medical care. Personal medical care is a very political issue for understandable reasons. First, when an individual is sick, they want care and help. Their need and misfortune elicit sympathy. Second, medical care is personal, immediate, and dramatic, whereas public health and other policy interventions are distant and abstract. Third, medical care providers, backed up by dramatic gains in science, own a strong brand and have pecuniary self-interest; they also have much political influence.

Allocating healthcare resources in the political process has some significant challenges. The most important risk is that individual medical care is, for practical purposes, a bottomless pit; demand is open-ended, so politicians will experience recurrent, unending pressures to deliver access to more and better services. Expenditures will escalate, and eventually, leaders will face significant opportunity costs and trade-offs with other priorities. It is never easy to limit or reduce services for a population. Such will be politically unpopular for a government that sets limits. It will take courageous leadership to rein in healthcare costs and gifted communication skills to explain it and still maintain the public's trust.

Funding Exceeding a Nation's Means Government spending is limited by national productivity. Fundamentally, all developed nations must succeed financially in the world economy. Michael Porter has described how this works in his book, *The Competitive Advantage of Nations*.[7] No country can survive for long when its growth in spending exceeds the increased productivity needed to earn the resources to pay for it. In this context, the middle- and high-income countries that we address in this workbook must come to see health not just as an expense and a desirable national benefit but also as a variable that contributes to or detracts from a nation's capacity to produce goods and services of value and thrive in a global economy. A healthy population can potentially enhance productivity and fund its costs. But the growing proportion of GDP spent on healthcare can constrain competitiveness. If productivity stagnates, a nation's resources to fund healthcare for all will decline.

The Inevitable Setting of Limits

Call it what you will—setting priorities, introducing limits, or rationing—reductions in collectively supported medical services are in our future. Through design improvements in their established health system, most developed nations can buy some time. But there is no time to waste in developing processes, practical approaches, and the ethics for setting limits.

Who Will Set Limits, and How? Our ability to set limits on medical expenditures has been a daunting challenge. In the public realm of support, we have established review mechanisms, often nongovernmental, to determine whether additional interventions are cost-effective. These guidelines work, to a degree. But if additional medical interventions yield even small marginal improvements, most people want them to be covered by their free or subsidized insurance or delivery system. At some point, then, setting limits (the withholding of coverage of interventions of small but nevertheless positive benefit) will be inevitable, at least in the basic programs of insurance or services available to all.

We have little research and few good examples of how best to ration services of low value. To date, we have scanty experience that guides us to effective and acceptable mechanisms to withhold care that has value, albeit small, to the individual.

The field of philosophy has identified some parameters of the solution. First, limit-setting should be seen as fair and reasonable Second, justice should be served by making decision-making transparent and open for review. Finally, John Rawls, the 20th century American liberal philosopher, introduced the concept of the "veil of ignorance", which suggests that decisions be displaced from the individuals at risk to a group that is detached from the problem. Nevertheless, we remain in the dark with regard to criteria for making decisions about limits to the benefits for which insurance should pay or for the capacity and benefits on offer in a universally available, publicly funded health system.

Healthcare systems have generally turned to the medical profession to set limits and thereby decide who gets what care. This has worked reasonably well in the past but is increasingly difficult to justify in the future. The criteria for doctors' decisions regarding referral or triage are largely implicit and inconsistent. Doctors are often put in a bind when asked to adjudicate whether a patient will receive a test or treatment of small but positive value. Are healthcare professionals stewards of the collective system or only answerable to the individual patient? The oath that doctors take explicitly puts the patient's interests first. Many doctors refuse to make rationing decisions that are needed for the sustainability of the insurance pool and the overall health of the population. The problem becomes even more fraught when doctors actually receive money for what appears to be withholding medical services of some, albeit little, benefit.

Ethicists should help us address the thorny issue of rationing. But the growing field of bioethics has largely sidestepped addressing the moral philosophy of setting limits. Yet bioethicists already deal with life and death decisions in healthcare. Now is the time for them to challenge themselves to create the principles and ethical framework to allocate scarce individual medical care resources.

The Role and Responsibility of Citizens It is unlikely that collective insurance can forever fully cover the costs of our collectively deteriorating health lifestyles, when these are actually the source of much of our current morbidity, mortality, and costs. Patients should do their part and fulfill their responsibilities in their own care as part of their medical team. Current medical attitudes that treat patients only as victims and not as agents of their own health are not sustainable. At the very least, we should recognize and reward good personal behavior in health habits and practices. Patients' responsible participation in their own health and illness management is as, or even more, important than the behavior of the providers of care.

Private Provision of Healthcare Services The need to set limits is inevitable only for collective insurance programs that share risk, whether public or private. However, as long as an individual pays the full costs of their care privately, there is no collective reason to limit their expenditure. Insurance coverage or the services themselves are no different from any other discretionary purchase. If individuals are willing to pay, they should be able to choose what they want, so long as there is prudent regulation to ensure high-quality medical care and avoidance of interventions that cause harm.

Some countries with publicly funded universal health insurance for medical care have already responded to the limits of the benefits and services they can afford to cover by allowing services to be purchased privately. Their national health insurance may limit access to some expensive · drugs or treatments of low effectiveness. Covered benefits, such as dental, mental, or social services, may be restricted even though the need remains.

Countries applying such restrictions often allow these services to be available to those who can afford them. They have allowed or even encouraged the formation of private insurance to top up the basic system. In these so-called two-tiered systems, individuals can choose to purchase additional insurance or pay directly for services and benefits that might not otherwise be covered in the universal scheme. People will inevitably make their own decisions about how to allocate their personal resources, and if one can afford these additional services, there should be no constraints except those related to safety and controlling dishonesty.

One such model, in England, demonstrates how private care can serve its national health system. The NHS requires that all individuals contribute financially to the basic insurance program through taxation and then must pay additionally for any services if they choose to opt out. The private service sector supports universal insurance in two ways: first, by contributing to it financially and, second, by freeing up capacity that the private payers do not use, thus increasing the capacity of public medical services. Despite its obvious challenge to the reality or perception of healthcare equality, the private system has yet to experience strong public disapproval from those who cannot afford it.

CONCLUSION

The benefits from well-designed health systems and provision of health-care services since WWII are indisputable. But storm clouds are gathering around the sustainability of these systems. Although the day of reckoning can be put off by interventions such as efficiency, effectiveness, and private opt-out measures, all collective insurance systems will ultimately reach a level of expenditure that will force them to set limits. Benefits are constrained by a ceiling effect that limits the system to a price that a nation or institution can afford. Inevitably, health for all will require some form of rational limitation of benefits, even with regard to some interventions that have value. The challenge for society, and bioethicists, is to understand these conflicts and guide how we decide to set limits.

Our view is that the issues of ethical rationing is the knottiest problem that will challenge national health systems in the future. That is, we need to answer the ethical, moral, political, and practical problems of saying "no" to a request for medical care of some level of benefit for the individual.

STUDY QUESTIONS

1. Most experts believe that public health interventions at the population level are more cost-effective in delivering health than individual medical care. What are the possible reasons that individual medical care is the larger investment in virtually all developed countries?
2. What effect would declining national productivity have on the delivery and financing of healthcare?
3. Why do you think that primary care doctor numbers are declining despite the repeated calls by the WHO and others for them to be the basis of all medical care?
4. What do you think is the most important accomplishment in medical care since WWII?
5. What does the history of the development of healthcare since WWII suggest about the most important goal(s) for planners of healthcare for the 21st century?

CHAPTER 4
Developing a Vision and Goals

For every complex problem there is an answer that is clear, simple, and wrong.
—H. L. Mencken

In this chapter, we lay out how to assess, define, and choose the vision and specific goals that your country will aspire to achieve through design of interventions in its health system. Why goals? It may be perplexing that we suggest that you start the change process by defining a vision and goals for your health system. Our natural instinct is to do something to fix a problem when it feels urgent. The reason for stepping back and considering goals is best summed up in a quip made by a revered American baseball player, Yogi Berra. He famously said, "You've got to be very careful if you don't know where you are going, because you might not get there." Without a realistic vision and honest goals, it is very difficult to know whether your interventions are actually improving your country's health system and getting it what it wants.

Setting strategic health goals is not an easy political task. Public opinion is bound to react to any setting of goals, except under the most trusted and communicative leadership in a mature, competent, and confident population. For that reason, most countries gloss over the specification of goals, concentrating instead on inputs to the system, hoping that these details adequately substitute for the outputs and outcomes.

Nevertheless, this book is about planning, and planners are responsible for thinking and developing a view about vision, goals and objectives. We want our students to understand how to think about health system goals and targets; without undertaking this process, no one is in a position to analyze whether planned and implemented changes have worked or not and what might be learned from their success or failure.

How should governments and political leaders make choices? The process for setting goals (and doing planning) benefits from a politically sheltered environment to do its work properly. The philosopher John Rawls attempted to deal with such difficult issues in distributive justice in his work in the 1970s.[1] Rawlsian philosophical theory is interesting to consider in a health context. Rawls contended that such decisions should be made behind a "veil of ignorance." This "veil" blinds people to facts and biases about themselves, so that their decisions are not tailored specifically to their own personal situation. The objective is to make difficult societal choices as though you did not know where in the social strata you might fall and how such decisions would affect you personally. Rawls believed that judgments made this way would be fairer. Rawls positioned his theory as hypothetical, as in practice it is nearly impossible for individuals to leave behind all their own lived experiences and biases.

At the most general level, global objectives and goals are not difficult to enumerate. The operating objectives for health system outputs comprise equity, effectiveness, efficiency, and responsiveness of the personal healthcare and public health services the health system provides. These outputs determine achievement of goals in relation to health system outcomes produced. Practically, these high level goals are fulfilled by maximizing the level and distribution of population health outcomes (such as life expectancy or premature mortality), managing well, protecting citizens from financial risk and thus providing universal access to health services, and producing high consumer satisfactions when the system is used. These goals should be achieved at a cost that is financially sustainable for the country.

A country's real challenge begins when it specifies exactly what these abstract goals mean in practice. Policymakers must define criteria for success, set priorities, and develop and apply specific policies in order to achieve health system goals with targets for the outputs and outcomes that the system delivers. These specifications are essential to the job of successfully managing health system functions (e.g., health system organization and governance, financing, and resource management), which are shaped by public attitudes and values about health and healthcare.

There are many ways to identify goals, objectives and targets for a health system. In some settings, political or business leaders can define and test such goals. Working from a position of strength and trust, a leader can speak candidly and sway the public to accept realistic expectations about goals. In other settings, a side process, sheltered from the public, may be necessary to reflect on the trade-offs and protect a winning but potentially unpopular strategic position. The former situation was in play, for example, in the Netherlands in the fertile period of the early millennial years when a goals-driven process led to a definition of national goals and objectives as well as some creative solutions. Public attitudes were such that the planners could forthrightly state that the preferred plan was financially unsustainable, and they forecast the need to address the criterion of affordability. However, continuing cost challenges persisted, and subsequently, the Netherlands implemented major reforms in 2006. These introduced regulated competition in a health system that was typically government-run. Their purpose was to improve efficiency, effectiveness, equity, and responsiveness of the health system and ensure sustainability.

A further approach used in priority-setting is the accountability for reasonableness (A4R) approach developed by ethicists (Box 4.1).[2] A4R does not identify the priorities for government investments; rather, it establishes the principles for a transparent process for legitimate public input in determining these priorities to guide investment decisions. The process explicitly articulates and links values and principles to decisions, outcomes, and goals. A4R identifies the principles that are relevant for policymakers and societies.[3] It has been used in several countries to aid decision-making. These include the United Kingdom, where the National Institute for Health and Clinical Excellence uses it to take social value judgments into account when recommending coverage for new treatments, and Mexico, where decisions about which diseases the social insurance schemes should cover were developed through engagement of such working groups to evaluate clinical, economic, ethical, and social considerations of policies.[4]

Box 4.1: ACCOUNTABILITY FOR REASONABLENESS

A4R is a process grounded in democratic principles aimed at legitimizing decision-making among "fair-minded" people who seek mutually justifiable terms of cooperation. A4R has four conditions [Ref]:

1. Publicity: Decisions that establish priorities in meeting health needs and their rationales must be publicly accessible.
2. Relevance: Policymakers should provide reasonable rationales that appeal to evidence, reasons, and principles accepted as relevant by

fair–minded people when justifying their decisions. Rationales should be relevant for a broad range of stakeholders in decision-making.
3. Revision and appeals: There must be mechanisms for challenge and dispute and, more broadly, opportunities for revision and improvement of policies in light of new evidence or arguments.
4. Regulation: There must be public regulation of the process to ensure that the first three conditions are met.

An expert-driven process can also be used. The Delphi technique[5] approach is a widely used method for goal-setting (we describe and use it later in this chapter). In this approach, a select group reviews alternatives, solicits expert opinions, studies and debates them, and then multivotes over several cycles to move systematically toward a consensus view.

ENVISIONING HEALTH SYSTEM GOALS AND OBJECTIVES

In this workbook, we are under no political constraints. Therefore, we attempt to follow a rather idealized evidence-based vision and goal-setting process, knowing that real-life situations in nations or businesses rarely can achieve this standard. As with any creative process, the path will not be clean or perfect. The aim of this chapter is to progress through semistructured steps and at the same time continuously reflect back to and readjust your tentative thoughts about vision, gaps, and goals. The end result will provide a foundation for your country group exercise in Chapter 5 of this volume to invent and agree to a working plan for a change in your selected country's health system.

Setting a vision, realistic goals, and targets for health is where system planning and design begin. Organized populations differ in their needs and means for health. Every population that comprises a health system has financial and capacity constraints and must set priorities. It is our natural instinct to feel that healthcare services should be directed at treating the sick and preventing illness. But that simple overview doesn't help much in setting priorities. One nation's vision and goals for health might be focused on increasing longevity, quality of life, and functionality of the elderly, while for another it could be on reducing the health factors that hamper the readiness of young people for education, work, and family development. Similarly, for business-based populations, the priority goal might not just be to improve longevity but also to maximize healthy lives to reduce absenteeism in its workforce and enable its highest productivity, while for another it might be to reduce medical care costs and increase its profitability.

The point is that there is no system that can respond to all needs, given everything that medical care and science has invented to intervene in health and illness. It is unlikely that any enterprise or nation can afford comprehensive insurance for all conditions and available interventions. Thus, it is a necessity that decision makers in any population design a system that reflects their priorities. The design of the health system must pursue the goals and objectives that the population wants to achieve.

Sizing Up How a Health System Works

An appropriate vision for change and useful goals entail matching aspirations with realistic assessments of how the system works. Setting up unrealistic, idealistic goals is of little use to planners. If the system is incapable of achieving them, the goals become a tease. Worse, expectations are created that undermine public trust in the system and those responsible for it.

Figuring out a country's health system's dynamics is essential for getting ready to intervene in it. Understanding more about how your system works in action is essential to figure out your objectives. The development of a vision and goals is a back and forth process of formulation, assessment, reaction, and improvement. The designer of goals needs a deepening understanding of their system's dynamics as well as its problems to tune its vision, figure out its objectives, and determine what to do and where, when, and how to do it.

In Chapter 2 of this volume, you produced a map of the constituent elements of your selected country's system. As you progress through the workbook, you will deepen your knowledge about how the system functions. This enables the health system designer to find the right thing to do at leverage points that maximize the probability of creating a virtuous cycle and minimize resistance when the system fights back. One needs to circle around a system and size things up. Our instincts most often entice us to point out a problem and directly attempt to fix it. Systems theory tells us that rarely works and often makes the problem worse.

Scoping out a system is an essential skill. The health system designer must become as good as possible at acquiring an understanding of how the system works as a whole to get the results it is producing. We also know that any redesign has uncertainty built into it. We cannot really predict what will happen, even with the best possible understanding of the way it works. An essential skill of system designers is to learn to watch how the system behaves. You must become good at listening to how the system responds in action, learning from this surveillance feedback and adapting quickly to emerging signals. Therefore, we need to approach change as an experiment in which we are open-minded observers and willingly ask whether and why our redesign is working.

Understanding the physiology of a functioning health system is challenging. First, in a complex system of interactions with positive (amplifying) and negative (balancing) feedback loops, predicting exact outcomes is not possible; knowing what to do is often beset with uncertainty. Second, systems are homeostatic and self-correcting. Therefore, they resist change and fight back. Third, there are time delays between cause and effect of an interaction. Finally, parts of the system are interconnected, so that interactions do not happen in isolation. The many interconnected and interdependent elements create extensive networks of feedback loops with variable time lags between the cause and effect of an action and nonlinear relationships between system elements, collectively creating *dynamic complexity*. An interaction in one part of the system influences other parts, generating a *system response* that is a result of the interactions among the system's elements rather than change in one element. Because of the dynamic complexity of health systems and the uncertainties inherent in changing it, the planner's skill and knowledge about how to push on a system is essential to create virtuous second-order change (rather than an unintended, deleterious consequence).

This workbook does not claim to make its users into expert diagnosticians of health systems. Many years of experience and learning are necessary to achieve such skills and expertise. However, we do hope to introduce different disciplines to the learner as they work through a real planning exercise and, by so doing, gain some experience with tools that might aid their understanding.

For those reasons, this chapter lays out a sequence of preparatory exercises that enable the designer to think about the system and its parts in a holistic way and from different perspectives. These aim to enable you to formulate an initial vision and pick your country's goals to change for improvement. These will facilitate the specific redesign of your system that you will undertake in Chapter 5 of this volume.

Exercises to Help You Develop a Sense of a System's Vision, Goals, and Objectives

The initial assignment in this chapter is to work on your own to gain a general understanding of your country's political and economic priorities and its vision and goals for health. The first exercises are to provide some semistructured guidance about reflecting on your system of care.

Doodling

Develop a rough sketch of your health system to a point where you could describe it in general terms and get others to comment and give feedback. Form a mental representation of your idea about how things work. Mental models can be made explicit by transforming them into push–pull flow diagrams. These enable one to express in graphic form how different pieces of a system interact and affect one another. Figure 4.1 is an example of a mental sketch to influence individual users to lower costs. Try to create such a diagram, showing graphically how the forces in your health system affect one another and how the design leads causally to health outcomes, satisfaction, and financial stability.

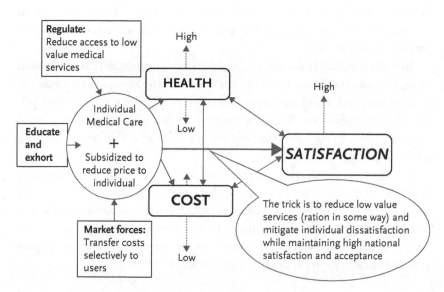

Figure 4.1 Sketch of an idea to control costs but maintain satisfaction.

Imagine how a leader in your country would describe his or her vision for what the system delivers. Some visions are vague ("Health for all by the year 2030"). Some countries have stated goals. Many are described in medical delivery terms, such as universal insurance coverage, evidence-based care decisions, and patient-centered care. Most descriptions are about process ("All citizens should have access to healthcare services") rather than outcomes ("All citizens will achieve a specified level of health").

These process goals often obscure what countries or enterprises really want. Taking a marketing perspective, we know that customers want to "hire" a product to do a job, or as legendary Harvard Business School marketing professor Theodore Levitt apparently used to tell his students "People don't want to buy a quarter-inch drill. They want a quarter-inch hole!"[cited in 6pxx] Ask yourself: Do people want a doctor or a test or a drug? What is it that they really want? The answer is likely to be to feel well, to forget that they are ill, to reduce their anxiety and worry, to live longer, to be reassured, to reduce pain, or to be able to function at the top of their mental or physical capacity.

Try to be more specific about what your country wants. Pick out at least one explicit statement related to the population's health status, individual financial risks, global satisfaction, or collective costs or affordability that will determine the sustainability of the system (Warning: This is hard to do). You might want to look at some attempts to do this exercise and see what you think. Here are two frameworks that have attempted to describe vision and functions.

1. Healthy People 2030 Framework
   https://www.healthypeople.gov/2020/About-Healthy-People/
   Development-Healthy-People-2030/Framework
2. National Health Service (NHS) Outcomes Framework
   https://digital.nhs.uk/data-and-information/publications/clinical-indicators/nhs-outcomes-framework/current#summary

An Exercise in Allocating Resources

All countries, businesses and organizations with responsibility for healthcare services must live within their means and yet carry out all of the functions of government including healthcare services. Because there are other national needs, not all of a country's resources can be allocated to healthcare. At any given level of expenditure, there are real trade-offs (opportunity costs) to diverting more of a nation's financial resources to deliver healthcare services.

In this exercise, think about the use of national resources. These include such programs as defense; education; public safety; infrastructure such as roads, rail, internet, and airports; environment; social support; income redistribution for the poor or old; tax collection; administration; justice; economic stabilization (inflation or depression); immigration; innovation; jobs; and economic development. Ask yourself what you think about the relative allocation in your country across all dimensions.

The exercise consists of making a list and assessing where resources need to be reallocated. Imagine that the government has no additional revenue to spend and new priorities require reductions somewhere else in the current pattern of allocation. The exercise should be to understand and compare the value that is added by each additional unit of expenditure. How does health fare in this process in your study country?

Formulating a Working Vision Statement

Vision statements are usually very general when they are used at all. Costs, affordability, or sustainability are rarely mentioned explicitly in vision statements. As an example, Healthy People 2030 (see previous link), the US vision developed in a government-sponsored planning process using expert panels and incorporated in the 2030 framework, is "A society in which all people can achieve their full potential for health and well-being across the lifespan."[7] A comparable vision statement for the English NHS in the past was "We strive to improve health and well-being and people's experiences of the NHS."[8] Neither includes a statement of constraints in prioritizing what the nation chooses to spend and can afford on healthcare services. Political considerations make it hard to publicize an honest vision; limitations or compromises are not popular.

We have a different purpose and reason for crafting a vision statement (and goals). This is intended to be a planners' tool, not a political statement. We believe that a realistic vision statement is an essential design element for planners and decision makers.

At this stage, we suggest that each student write down a draft vision statement for their country. Try to make it realistic; a vision with no constraints, trade-offs, or limits is a weak or even useless planning tool. Be specific. Some of you may find that a vision has already been selected, which is a starting point for the country. Write it down. Others may need to reflect on their personal responses to the earlier chapters and exercises and invent one that seems to be the best fit for their nation. This should describe what you, in private, believe your nation's health system should realistically aspire to be.

Drilling Down on Goals and Objectives

In this section of homework, each student will follow a semistructured format to develop specific details about the capability (strengths and weaknesses) and context (opportunities and threats) that the existing system in their study country faces. At this preliminary stage, students are not required to state objective evidence for their choice; the exercise solicits an impressionistic view based on the work the students have done so far and the hunches they are developing. However, we do encourage students to access literature references to support and buttress the case for their choices, which they may be called upon to present when the group meets later in this chapter.

SWOT Analysis

SWOT analysis is a commonly used tool in strategic planning. It serves to identify internal and external conditions that influence the health system. SWOT analysis helps identify what could be further enhanced (strengths), what needs to be improved (weaknesses), what to capitalize on (opportunities), or what to prepare for (threats). The SWOT process identifies opportunities and threats by examining the broad context to ascertain external factors that are influencing the health system, such as demographic and epidemiological changes, sociocultural norms, political factors, or technological advancement. Strengths and weaknesses of the system are recognized through analysis of health system performance against its own set goals and objectives or by comparison to the set goals or performance drawn from other systems.

SWOT is to be used as a tool in the early stages of decision-making processes. This analysis can inform the goals and objectives in a health system. SWOT helps in the creation of an action plan by identifying elements needed to launch a change process and then uses that information to identify the best route for change. SWOT analysis is widely used by organizations, whether for a business venture, a project, or personnel development.[9]

SWOT analysis helps to answer questions in the following four categories to generate background information about the existing and anticipated environment. The name is an acronym for the parameters the technique examines:

- *Strengths*: What are the strongest and most valuable features of the health system as it is now?
- *Weaknesses*: What current conditions of the system weaken its potential for change? Weaknesses, like strengths, are inherent features of your health system as it is now, so focus on its current results, shared values, workforce, resources, systems, and procedures.
- *Opportunities*: What conditions in the external context can create a favorable setting and could best be exploited to improve the system?
- *Threats*: What changing factors in the external context could cause trouble for the health system now or in the future?

In our use of the tool in Tables 4.1 and 4.2, we will apply SWOT first to generate observations about our target health system. *Individual students should fill in each of the four quadrants with their responses. They should be prepared to make the case for their choices in their group class.*

Table 4.1 STRENGTHS AND WEAKNESSES

SWOT Analysis: 1–2 sentences each point. Put points roughly in descending priority order.	
Strengths: Ways in which your health system excels. What are its unique resources and strengths? What do outside experts admire most?	Weaknesses: Ways in which your system is weak. Where does it need to improve? What areas need more resource? What do experts view as your system's greatest deficiency?

Table 4.2 OPPORTUNITIES AND TREATS

SWOT Analysis: 1–2 sentences each point. Put points roughly in descending priority order.	
Opportunities: Conditions exploitable for improvement. What trends in the external context might facilitate change? Are there obvious opportunities that could be harnessed?	Threats: What changes in external factors could destabilize your current health system?

Thinking About Gaps: The Spider Diagram

Your preparation for the group meeting is to reflect on your assessment of strengths and weaknesses, first to use it as an input to assess the current performance of your system. Second, you will use it to speculate about where it should be in the future using a spider diagram (also referred to as a radar diagram). The spider diagram is a tool that facilitates comparing existing and desired future performance of a system across categories of performance measurement. The spider diagram framework identifies performance categories and visual displays ratings of the selected performance categories.

The spider diagram exercise is intended to rate performance across different functional parameters. The ratings are to be evidence-based to the degree possible. However, the planner may have to estimate performance intuitively where data do not exist. It is said that the measurable often drives out the important; that is certainly true in health. The absence of data does not relieve the planner from the responsibility of making assessments.

The basic spider diagram is shown in Figure 4.2. We have selected 12 performance parameters that are commonly used in cross-system

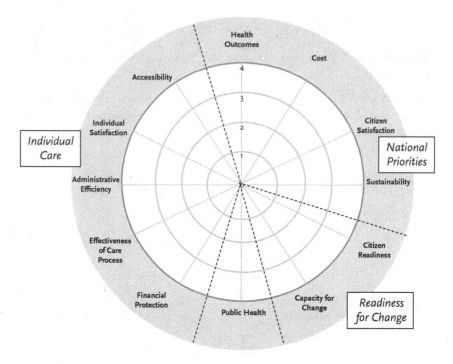

Figure 4.2 Spider diagram of 12 performance measurement areas.
Key: Ratings are 0 for no activity, 1 for poor, 2 for fair, 3 for good, and 4 for excellent performance.

comparisons, supplemented by a few measures of the degree of need and the capacity for change, neither of which is generally formally measured. There are data sources for many of these categories.

Some common measures follow in Box 4.2, where each of the 12 parameters is described, and we give suggestions about criteria for measuring the 12 performance categories in economically highly developed countries. Many sources such as the World Bank, Organisation for Economic Cooperation and Development (OECD), World Health Organization and the Commonwealth Fund generate reports of health system performance and have published comparative data using available tools. These are listed in Box 4.2. In some areas of performance measurement, no specific data are available, but estimations can still be made subjectively and impressionistically. We ask that you make these assessments and also think about how you might measure this function if you had the resources to do so.

Box 4.2: SUGGESTED MEASURES FOR THE 12
PERFORMANCE CATEGORIES

National priorities

- Health outcomes: What is the level of health in the nation overall?
  - Average life expectancy at birth or from other age such as 30 or 60
  - Burden of illness: DALY, QALY
  - Well-being—healthy life years
  - Measures of functionality
  - Avoidable illness
- Costs: Is the nation getting its money's worth?
  - Total healthcare expenditure
  - %of GDP spent on healthcare
  - % health expenditure/GDP: % of GDP compared to other countries
  - Allocative efficiency: producing the right outputs to achieve goals (i.e., the mix of services to maximize health outcomes and user satisfaction for available resources)
  - At the macroeconomic level, health expenditure as a % of GDP
  - Technical efficiency (e.g., % of health expenditure spent on administering the system, average cost per hospital stay, or average length per hospital stay for acute admission)
- Citizen satisfaction: How does a nation regard its health system—satisfied, proud, dissatisfied?
  - Self-rating approval levels of national system (Commonwealth Fund)
  - Would you give your country a first, second, or a third place for its health system?
- Sustainability of national healthcare services
  - Total healthcare expenditure
  - % of GDP spent on healthcare
  - % health expenditure/GDP: % of GDP compared to other countries
  - % of annual national budget spent on healthcare
  - Does national productivity growth support expansion of expenditures?
  - What is the affordability of the health system to the nation, given trade-offs with other important national investments?
  Readiness for change and the public health system
- Citizen readiness: The level of demand for change in the system
  - National dissatisfaction
  - Political and health literacy
  - Engagement with the issue

- National capacity for change: The capacity for making significant change in the system
  - Leadership strength
  - Decision-making process capable of overcoming an impasse or stalemate and coming to an agreement
  - Capital availability
  - Political alignment around need for health change
  - Political agreement around the key change leverage points
    - Strong tools for driving change such as use of regulation or market forces
    - Ability to get things done once a decision is made
    - Can the system measure its progress, respond to problems, and improve itself?
- Public health: The capacity, functionality, and readiness of the public health sector to contribute to health and healthcare services
  - National health education
  - Public policy influence
  - Readiness for evolving health emergencies
  - Health surveillance and data management
  - Safety standards
  Individual healthcare services
- Effectiveness off care process: the extent to which a desired outcome is achieved when a cost-effective intervention is applied to a population. Often thought of as *quality*.
  - % investment in cost-effective interventions (e.g., prevention, World Health Organization best buys for noncommunicable diseases, interventions included in Disease Control Priorities 3)
  - % expenditure or rate of inappropriate interventions (e.g., Caesarean sections)
  - Investment in cost-effective domains: % public health costs/health expenditure
  - Use of evidence-based guidelines
  - How safe and reliable is care as measured by
    - Malpractice levels
    - Preventable errors
- Administrative efficiency: the healthcare delivery system's ability to produce service outputs at minimum costs
  - Average hospital expenditure or length of stay for treatment of acute MI
  - Average hospital length of stay
  - Hospital beds per 1,000 population and % occupancy
  - Ratio of GPs to hospital specialists
  - Patients' adherence to recommended and prescribed treatments
  - Integration, communication, and coordination of care
  - Administrative efficiency (% health expenditure spent on administration)

- Equity (financial protection to enable healthcare for all)
  - Fairness in allocation of resource or services to different individuals or groups
  - Accessibility of different individuals or groups to needed services
    - Waiting times for first appointment
    - Variation in rates of use of evidence-based treatments by group
  - Unmet need
  - Individual financial protection
    - Affordability: The degree to which the level of subsidy makes care affordable for an individual
- Responsiveness (individual satisfaction) of users' legitimate needs and expectations
  - User surveys
    - Does the care meet expectations of service quality?
    - Do users feel empowered?
    - Is the care responsive and timely?
    - Reliable, dependable, and predictable?
    - Trustworthy and confidence-generating?
    - Service-oriented, engaging and sensitive to patient needs and preferences?

Abbreviations: %, percentage; DALY, disability-adjusted life years; GDP, gross domestic product; GP, general practitioner; MI, myocardial infarction; QALY, quality-adjusted life years.

As examples, Figures 4.3 and 4.4 show spider/radar diagram examples for the United Kingdom and the United States, reflecting general assessments that we have put together for the two countries. The United Kingdom has baseline scores that are generally high, reflecting its low cost, universal accessibility, and high national regard. Its largest gap points to the goal of improving public health and health outcomes, but we also believe that the overall healthcare system is underfunded; our goal statement would focus on increasing funding with a focus on cost-effective initiatives that enhance public health measures and improve patient outcomes.

The US spider diagram shows generally lower performance reflecting its high costs, variable accessibility, and mixed clinical outcomes. We have selected its largest gap to be in value, reflecting its high expenditure and yet middling national health. Public health capacity enhancement would be another priority. Both must be improved, either by reducing costs, reallocating resources, or improving health outcomes. Without a redesign to reduce costs, American healthcare services will become less accessible, less fair and equitable even than now, and with worsening health overall. Solidarity will be under even greater threat.

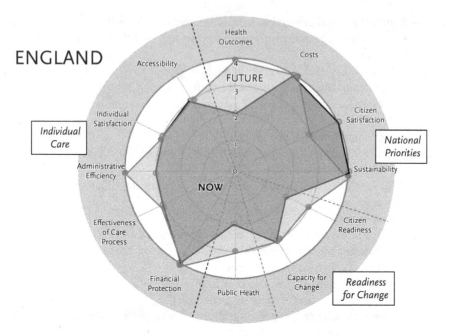

Figure 4.3 Spider diagram for England's health system.

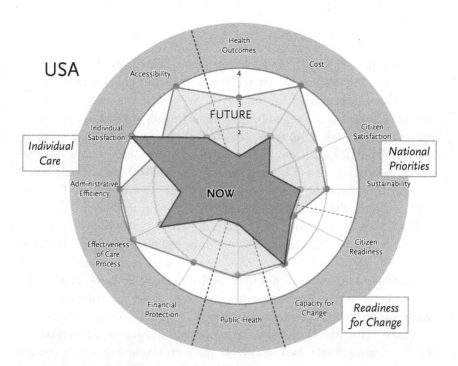

Figure 4.4 Spider diagram for the US health system.

Assignment

Premeeting

Before the group meeting, each student should rate their system as it is operating today. You are responsible for taking tentative positions about your country's current and future performance. Based on your rough model of how your system works, analysis of the external context (opportunities and threats), and estimation of strengths and weaknesses of the health system, you should assign ratings using your spider diagram. You should transcribe your ratings onto the blank spider diagram (Figure 4.2) and connect the dots. These performance ratings, where possible, should be based on actual country evidence as measured and reported in specific studies. Useful references are listed in Table 4.3.

Your responses will be the basis for group discussion. In the group meeting, you will work in your country teams to review what each of you has proposed and to reach agreement about your group's spider/radar diagram. Individual student responses to the preparatory assignment questions are important inputs to the group's learning.

Table 4.3 USEFUL SOURCES FOR ASSESSING HEALTH SYSTEM PERFORMANCE

World Bank: Health, Nutrition and Population Statistics	http://datatopics.worldbank.org/health/
World Bank: World Development Indicators—Health Systems	http://wdi.worldbank.org/table/2.12
OECD Health Statistics	http://www.oecd.org/els/health-systems/health-data.htm
OECD Health at a Glance	http://www.oecd.org/health/health-systems/health-at-a-glance-19991312.htm
OECD Reviews of Health Systems	https://www.oecd.org/els/health-systems/reviews-health-systems.htm
OECD Health Reports by Country	http://www.oecd.org/health/bycountry/
OECD Health Care Quality and Outcomes	https://www.oecd.org/health/health-systems/health-care-quality-and-outcomes.htm
Commonwealth Fund: International Health Care System Profiles	https://www.commonwealthfund.org/international-health-policy-center/system-profiles

Abbreviation: OECD, Organisation for Economic Cooperation and Development.

Next, you should commit to where levels of performance in each of the 12 domains ought to stand in their system in the medium term, say, in 10 years. Choose those places (up to three) where you believe that closing the gap (between current performance and where your system needs to get to in the future) will lead to the greatest improvement. These results should be mapped onto your spider diagram.

Priorities must be set among the gaps that emerge between current and future performance. *You are to rank order the three most important gaps between where the system is now and where you feel it needs to be. You should be prepared to present your argument about why you have chosen these three and your rationale for the order of ranking.*

Country Group Meeting

This small group meeting will cover three linked activities. The group will

1. *Collectively review their identified strengths and weaknesses followed by opportunities and threats;*
2. *Present, discuss, and integrate their spider diagrams and gaps analysis and consolidate their choices; and*
3. *draft a single group vision statement and goals for their country.*

These activities could take place in a morning or afternoon session that completes all three tasks, or a course leader could separate the group exercises and schedule sessions to deal individually with the three learning activities, thereby making it possible to break up and spread out the homework assignment.

1. *Ranking strengths and weaknesses, opportunities and threats.* First, the assembled group will present and discuss each participant's three most important proposed strengths and weaknesses from the SWOT analysis. Our suggestion is that each student be asked to list on the board their top two responses of strengths and weaknesses and explain briefly the reasons for their choices. When all answers have been listed on a whiteboard, a group session leader leads the group in consolidating duplicate answers. Once all the student responses have been presented and the group has conducted a round of questions, answers, and justifications, the group will then further condense the list using a simple multivoting technique. The process is repeated for all four SWOT categories.

2. *Multivoting:* This is a relatively straight-forward process to organize student discussion in assessing and consolidating choices among each of the four categories in their SWOT analysis. This is most simply done by

asking each student to identify their top three choices in the category and to assign a 3 for their top, 2 for the second, and 1 for their third choice. The leader adds the scores next to each strength (and, separately, each weakness, opportunity, and threat), generating a rough rank ordering of all responses.

The ranked listing of strengths and weaknesses will be used next in this chapter in an exercise to identify gaps and thereafter to select high level goals to present to the entire group. The threats and opportunities answers will be used in the next chapter as an input to the work of identifying the most important externalities that will influence the change that the team proposes for their country to deliver their selected goals and objectives.

3. *Agreeing on the baseline spider diagram:* The group will determine their collective rating for each parameter, progressing one by one through all 12. Each parameter of current performance is listed on the board. Each student rating is listed next to the designated performance measure. Only those students whose responses lie outside that of the main cluster are asked to defend their choice. Individuals silently rerank, and their new responses are listed. The highest total determines the rating on the spider diagram for that parameter. When all 12 parameters are complete, the leader draws the final baseline spider diagram on the board. All prior scores for the 12 parameters are erased.

4. *Setting future targets:* Reviewing the list of prioritized strengths and weaknesses and the baseline spider diagram on a nearby board, the students silently consider their premeeting choices about future priorities and revise their rankings. They then repeat the process of determining their group's collective rating for each parameter and chart the results on their baseline spider diagram. The difference in ranking between the group's baseline and the individual student's designated future performance goal equals each student's designation of the gap on each of the 12 parameters. Each group member silently selects and ranks their top three priorities about which gaps are most important to fix.

5. *Prioritizing gaps in a Delphi technique exercise:* Before digging in deeper, your group will want a way to understand what members are thinking as they attempt to reach general agreement in the group. By this time, you and most of your colleagues in your study group have developed your own general idea about what you think needs to be changed or fixed in your target country. A useful exercise to collectively set priorities is the Delphi technique.

We will use the Delphi technique as if you were a group of experts meeting to agree on your nation's priorities for change. The Delphi technique is a method of group decision-making and prediction that involves

Health status	3-gtm, 2-lst, 2-ria, 3-jm, 2-rtt	12
National cost	2-lst, 3-rmf	5
Citizen satisfaction	2-gtm	1
Sustainability	2-ria, 3-jm, 2-rtt	7
Citizen readiness	2-lst	2
National capacity for change	2-gtm	2
Productivity from health		
Individual financial protection	3-jm, 2-rtt, 2-ria	7
Carrying out the care process		
Administrative efficiency	2-ria	2
Individual satisfaction		
Accessibility		

Figure 4.5 Prioritizing student choices of priority gaps.

successive multivoting following waves of structured discussion in which the judgments of participants (usually experts) are shared before each vote. It was invented at the Rand Corporation in the 1950s for maximizing the validity of group predictions and decisions.

The work group leader asks for individual gap preferences each has chosen as their three most important targets from among the 12 parameters. These should be ranked as a 3 (top), 2, or 1 (lowest priority) with the priority written next to the chosen parameter and with the student's initials next to their choices. The scores are summed. An example is shown in Figure 4.5.

The group will review all 12 categories one by one. Each student has identified the 3 of the 12 gaps that reflect their main concerns, and discusses their reasoning when the appropriate parameter comes up. They present their justification and explain their thinking about why they have chosen that gap as a target. What makes the Delphi technique unique is that when participants have completed all 12 categories, they are given the chance to modify their choices and rankings after hearing the justification of others' choices. If there is significant shifting, another round (or more) of change and defense is followed up by summarizing scores and reviewing the top five or so as a group. The outliers are asked to speak persuasively about the reasons they have persisted; their objective should be to persuade the others to support their position. The process ends with a rank-ordered list of priority gaps.

6. *Articulating goals:* The group's next task is to take its identified gaps and reconstitute them as 10-year goals. As a collective exercise, the group restates the top five or so gaps as goals. To map future goals, the group will return to the 10-year goals they identified in their preparatory self-study but this time take into account the opportunities and threats analysis that

identifies the factors that will impact on the health system in the future. Do the goals still seem appropriate? Students will undertake the same process of self-reflection, followed by an open discussion process. Identifying goals makes clearer what the redesign to be formulated in Chapter 5 of this volume has to accomplish. The rankings should be modified and the spider diagram redrawn to show the targeted future performance.

7. *Closing in on vision, gaps, and goals:* In their final activity in this exercise, the group should tune the working vision and the priority problems. You have three inputs to integrate and align: your vision statement, your collective gap analysis as informed by your agreed strengths and weaknesses, and a formulation of specific gaps and goals to be achieved. At this stage, the group should briefly discuss, at a high level, the feasibility of the goals. Do a reality test to see if the vision and goals, resources, and change environment are reasonably enough aligned for you to feel optimistic about your capacity to find and initiate design changes that might work. To be sure, all these steps are subjective, perhaps more impressionistic and instinctive than you might hope.

The point of this goal-setting exercise is to understand the challenge from different perspectives, not to arrive at a definitive answer. At this stage in the process, we would suggest that groups consider their rank ordering of goals as preliminary. These goals will be the starting point for your work in Chapter 5 and later chapters of this volume—when you will come up with specifically what to do to achieve your goals. The purpose of this activity is for designers to understand, as best as possible, what they are trying to do and hoping to accomplish. Being able to describe the end game also establishes an explicit target that makes it possible to assess the degree to which the design has achieved its proposed system improvements.

The final step in this chapter is for the working group to create a coherent and consistent statement of purpose that integrates vision, gaps, and goals. Taking a step back and a deep breath, the group should undertake a general discussion starting with a review of the vision, strengths and weaknesses, and goals to see if its selections feel coherent and appropriate. Ask "What do I like about this vision and our goals?" "What do I dislike or am I worried about?"

At the most basic level, you want your vision and priorities to make sense. Is your vision reasonable, given all you know about your country? Is it the right vision? Can you justify it? Do your priority goals align with your vision? If you concentrated on improving performance in these areas, would you be closer to achieving your vision?

Another useful exercise is to create an elevator pitch. The idea is that if you were on an elevator with a high-level decision maker, you might have a minute or two to respond to a question such as "What is your view about where our health system should be heading?" You want to be ready. Members of the group could formulate an elevator pitch and practice delivering it to the group.

Formulating the health system's vision, goals, and objectives for their country is neither easy nor, frankly, completed at this point. It is difficult to prescribe a creative process. There is also no right or wrong answer. One never knows when an insight will suddenly pop up and open a new way of thinking about goals and system changes to achieve them. As we go through the remaining chapters of this workbook, the system thinker will constantly be cycling back and forth between ideas and goals and vision, asking questions, and remaining open to new insights and changes to their approach.

We believe that the designer can be helped in this self-reflective process by returning to fundamental questions probing the *what, why, when, where,* and *how* of goal formulation and design policies or interventions. Here are several questions that have been useful to us over the years:

- What difference will attaining this goal or target make?
- What problem(s) is this solution intended to solve?
- If things went really well, what results would we see?
- What are the measures of success for each problem you are targeting? How would you know that your proposed policy or intervention is working?
- Is there alignment between the vision and the proposed gaps?
- Strategy is about making choices; what choices have we rejected in coming up with this one?
- What are the downside risks to look out for? What is the worst thing that could happen if this goes wrong?
- Is achieving our vision or goals feasible?

Deliverables

Each group will write a two-page double-spaced summary of what they propose as a vision and the three or four most appropriate health goals (targets for change) for the country they are studying. The summary will include a brief description of their specific rationale/justifications/reasons for their choices—not just what they propose as vision and goals, but also why they propose them, and if the goals were achieved, what would be their impact on the vision and the country's health system.

CHAPTER 5

Developing Plans for Change

A Framework for Designing a High-Value Health System

It ain't what you don't know that gets you into trouble. It's what you know for sure that just ain't so.

—Mark Twain

INTRODUCTION TO WHAT THE STUDENTS WILL DO

This chapter's objective is for your work group to produce one system intervention plan (SIP) for your country. In the earlier chapters, you learned the components of a health system, identified the common underlying system problems many health systems share, took a stab at constructing the vision and goals of the health system in your specific country, and made a tentative start at identifying gaps that need closing to achieve these goals. In this chapter, you will attempt to discern the weak points ready for change and discover the interventions that could make the system function better.

This chapter will present various techniques and exercises to help you find interventions that work. The process you will go through is designed to generate a solution to fix your chosen system performance gap. The chapter presents a semi-structured design process for working from goals to means to build an intervention plan. The participants in each country-specific small group will follow a structure and process model to identify and propose an intervention to achieve the goals, objectives, and targets they have selected for their chosen country in Chapter 4 (see Box 5.1).

Box 5.1: SMALL GROUP ACTIVITIES

Your group activities are to

1. Understand the problems and causes underlying the goals the group selected as its target in Chapter 4 of this volume.
   a. Make a good diagnosis of the reasons for underperformance of your health system.
   b. Using your existing base of knowledge, analyze the root causes of the targeted gaps.
2. Generate an SIP for achieving the goal.
   a. Using a semi-structured process, generate a broad array of possible intervention ideas.
3. View the ideas that each small group member has developed.
   a. Present your proposed SIP to your colleagues in the group.
   b. Critique each other's SIP proposals. Each student will be the primary reviewer on another student's proposed SIP.
4. Decide the best intervention for your small workgroup to implement in your selected country.
   a. Discuss your group's different ideas.
   b. Prioritize and select one SIP to stress test, refine, and improve in Chapter 6 of this volume.
5. Create a succinct draft description of your plan to present and justify your choice to other course participants in a large group meeting.

Getting Started

General Issues in Designing and Making Improvements in a National Health System

Finding the best interventions and the right place to start is not easy. To maximize your chance of success in these areas, you need to approach this design phase holistically. That is, as you and your group generate and test ideas for change, you must keep the whole system continuously in mind to assess the intended and unintended consequences of your proposed design interventions. With this perspective, you may discover—and should be open to—revising even your initial vision and selected goals on which your group has chosen to work. This process of creating an intervention should be iterative, examining whole-system effects of the proposed interventions as you progress with your design. You should seek ideas that expand your thinking before narrowing down and selecting a few things to change.

We use the same word "system" to mean both a product and a process. In this chapter, you will create a system improvement plan, which we refer to as a SIP. The process for analyzing and developing your system improvement plan (SIP) is called *systems improvement planning* to distinguish it from the process of *quality improvement* (QI), or continuous improvement. We described the method of systems thinking in Chapter 1. In our view, creating an SIP deploys a "systems thinking" approach to the initial phase of designing a system intervention (identifying a problem, understanding its root causes, and planning design interventions). We consider QI to be the process of doing successive plan–do–check–act cycles during implementation to assess, fix, and optimize the components of a quality improvement intervention in a system. You will have a chance to apply QI later, in Chapter 6, as one of the process tools used to test and improve your SIP.

In this chapter, we present system improvement planning as a whole health system design process not just limited to healthcare delivery interventions. In the last chapter, you were asked to set a vision, goals, and targets for change in a full health system, including goals not only directed at existing healthcare service but also to other system elements that influence the health of a nation. As shown in Figure 1.1 in Chapter 1 of this volume, a health system is more than healthcare delivery services such as individual medical care and public health. A health system includes other elements that affect the health of a nation. These include influences such as citizen's personal health behaviors, social determinants of health like pollution and the economy, and even our mental maps and beliefs about life and death.

In improving a health system, designers have a wide range of general options. These range from the most straightforward fixes to the most radical interventions. Remember that every system is limited. Each is able, even in its most perfect expression, to deliver only the results that their basic design is capable of producing. And no real-life system is perfectly efficient and effective; every system needs management and tuning to achieve its full design potential. Therefore, the simplest category of improvement is that which enables an existing health system design to run better. System reinvention offers a radical improvement alternative at the other extreme of the spectrum. A system designer can change the fundamental system design model, aspiring to transform and change its very rules and constraints.

Creativity

Creative problem-solving draws on many approaches and skills. There are at least two general ways of thinking to come up with a plan to improve a healthcare system. The first methodology is deductive. The planner focuses on improving an existing system through an analytically driven step-by-step process. This approach uses tools such as business management, balance sheets and budgets, project management, the application of production improvement methods such as statistical process control as in Six Sigma or short-cycle quality improvement, research methods based on scientific evidence to determine what works best, measurement of performance, and education and training. All these tools are important, especially in getting the most efficiency, effectiveness, equity, responsiveness, and customer service and satisfaction out of an existing system.

The second approach to creative thinking can be thought of as inductive. One can't plan for it logically. The ideas spring into awareness out of some intuitive disruption of structured thinking based on existing models. In this approach, the process breaks away from the existing assumptions and rules; the designer breaches the limitations of an existing system design to create something new. The result is to change something about the basic system structure itself. In this process, all the elements of an existing or a green-field system are up for reshaping. Because the given system itself is interactive and dynamic, the planner is facing a problem of greater complexity. Inductive thinking makes it hard at first to know what to do and exactly where and when to intervene. Moreover, it is difficult to predict outcomes when one embarks on an intervention. Here the aim is one in which the creative process is open, unknown, and not amenable to the application of learned disciplines.

Both approaches are useful. There are many deductive methodologies that can be used to improve a health system. We expect our audience to learn how and where to apply these tools situationally and well. However, our special hope is to elicit inductive thinking by stimulating creativity tools that encourage out-of-the-box thinking. We hope our readers will learn new ways to overcome the inherent design limitations that restrict change in any current health system and to model new structures that create a new systems dynamic.

The Learning Plan

Individual Assignment

Each small group member will first undertake the improvement planning exercise on their own. Everyone will work with the priority goal identified for your country in the last chapter. The text will guide you through a process.

The initial activity is to conceive of and formulate a first draft of a feasible intervention to attain the selected goals from Chapter 4. Your assignment is to produce a draft SIP. Your draft SIP should be written up in proposal style. You will work on the following steps: review your and the group's vision, gap, and all goals; restate the chosen gap and goal in your own terms; create one or more interventions; describe your proposed system intervention in general terms; specify the specific problem your intervention will solve if everything goes well; answer the "So what? Who cares?" question of why it is important and what difference it would make; list and explain all the causal steps in the intervention pathway along with their expected results; and provide sufficient detail of the measures of success at each step to enable an observer to know if the target was successfully achieved. In the next session we present a process to guide you through defining and then designing the interventions at each causal step in your SIP.

There will be two meetings of your country group. The goal for the first meeting is for each student to present their draft SIP proposal and be given critical assessment. Before the meeting, you should circulate an electronic copy of your SIP to all fellow students in your country group. You are expected to read SIP proposals of all the others in your country group. Each group member should have been assigned as the reviewer of the SIP from one fellow student. The critical review of a colleague's SIP is your homework assignment to be carried out twice: once before the first meeting and a second review of the revised SIP prior to the second group meeting.

At your first work group meeting, each student will present his or her own and critique one other student's proposal. Each presentation will follow the standardized SIP format described in the following discussion (Box 5.2). The format should be applied to each step in the causal pathway between initiating the change and meeting the target(s) that delivers your selected goal. The reviewer should summarize what they liked (strengths) and what needs improvement (weaknesses) for each step. The objective of this first review meeting is to provide feedback to the presenter about what they can do to improve their SIP intervention so that they can ready their proposal for presentation at the second small group meeting.

1. The health system gap and the problem it creates
   - Description of the system gap your plan intends to fix and the goal you intend to achieve.
   - Significance: why this problem is important to fix; its adverse impact on citizens, providers, insurers, payers, and the system?
   - Your analysis of factors that create and exacerbate the problem you have selected.
2. The intervention
   - Your proposed intervention(s).
   - What is its expected impact?
   - What is the causal chain between your intervention and the outcome(s) that will solve your priority problem (this should be shown in graphic form)?
3. Intervention options considered
   - Why do you think this solution would be the most effective in solving the priority problem?
4. The benefits of the proposed intervention
   - What is the impact on the group's vision for the country?
   - The expected benefits of fixing the problem in terms of performance outcomes, costs, equity, individual patient satisfaction, collective satisfaction, provider capacity, and political impact.
   - How would you know that you have reached your intervention target? List the measures.
   - Describe the measures you will recommend using to assess the impact of your intervention on the ultimate goal of the SIP.
   - If possible, indicate how long it would take to earn back the costs of development and the likely change in revenues and/or other outcomes that might result from implementing your proposal.
5. Implementation risks that need to be mitigated
   - Does the proposal seem feasible?
   - What is the expected expense of implementation? Are there downside risks (what could go wrong and what would be the consequences?). Include your preliminary assessment of system costs and sustainability, national acceptability, and any likely change in the cost to the patient.

The second period of self-study is to modify your SIP based on reflection and feedback and to redraft and prepare it for a final presentation to your same country work group. During this process, you will assign your proposal to a yield (benefit)/effort, 2 × 2 table to categorize your SIP and use that perspective as a way to improve the plan and/or lower its cost and effort.

Understanding the Deliverable

The primary output from this chapter is the development of an SIP. The core of the plan is the proposed intervention by which the *status quo* of your country system and specific problem area is transformed into an output that produces the goal you and, later, your group identify. The intervention is a change process, represented as the sequence of steps to proceed from the beginning to the end result. The linking between the steps is referred to as a *causal chain*. Each step in a causal chain produces a result that is the input to the next step as shown in Figure 5.1. The steps are linked in a sequential change process that delivers the result.

Producing a draft of your SIP is the output of this independent study process. The format of the final SIP is laid out in Box 5.2. The write-up is short and intended to focus on facilitating a review of the goals, problem, and your ideas for an intervention to improve health in your country. However, the proposal should be detailed enough to enable you and your colleagues to decide about taking it to its next step in development to create a detailed SIP that can be implemented. A pictorial representation of your causal chain is essential. Usually, the plan is about two pages or less in length and follows a relatively standardized format, consisting of a summary of the problem, a description of the proposed idea, and the answers to several common concerns. These include what benefits might result, what risks there might be, how much it will cost, and what likely return (payback in better health) might be expected. At this first self-study stage, where you are still generating and prioritizing ideas, we suggest you use the SIP format in your group as a template to compare and contrast your intervention ideas thus far.

This two-page document will be a test of your and, later, your group's success in selecting a problem, identifying and understanding its root causes, and of how powerful your proposed intervention(s) will be in addressing these root causes and delivering upon your goal for a change. This step of writing is critical to understanding and powerfully presenting your analysis and argument. In settings where a

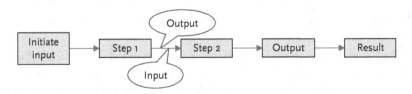

Figure 5.1 A causal chain to deliver an intervention.

decision must be made about investing resources, you would be expected to make your case concisely and to be able to defend your proposal logically and persuasively. In contrast to academic settings, where individuals are often willing to wade through long documents, decision makers (including policymakers, doctors, or managers) want proposals to be short, focused, and punchy.

As an aside, learning to write such a proposal can be a worthwhile skill. Whether your career entails policymaking, clinical practice, research, administration, or other types of leadership, you will frequently find yourself making plans, proposing ideas, and arguing for their implementation. This type of format can be useful in organizing your thoughts and strengthening your presentation in such cases.

DESIGNING THE INTERVENTION

An intervention can take many forms. It could be a relatively simple correction of a straightforward problem of inefficiency, ineffectiveness, inaccessibility, or poorly provided service; on the other hand, your intervention may need to fix breakdowns in a complex, dynamic system displaying vague symptoms, inadequate information, or unclear causes of dysfunction. The former problems lend themselves to standard forms of analysis— run charts, accounting and audit reports, patterns of use, complaints, and market surveys—and deductive methods of diagnosing and fixing the problem. The latter are wicked problems to understand and solve. In these cases of dynamic complexity, root causes are difficult to discern, and interventions are fraught with high uncertainty about whether and, if so, how they will work.

There are no magic formulas for thinking of a high-value intervention. Crafting a change to fix a complex problem cannot be standardized, mechanized, or routinized. The process is iterative, often intuitive, and involves ongoing learning. It usually requires inductive as well as deductive thinking and reasoning. No one knows exactly how one comes up with creative, effective ideas or interventions, although many consulting firms purport to know the best process. In the absence of research evidence to identify best practices, you are free to select any process that works for you and your group.

Fortunately, the common approaches to generate ideas are helpful with diverse problems, complexity, and improvement interventions. Developing a deep understanding of the underlying causes of the problem under study is universally a good first step. Loose–tight structured problem-solving can generate ideas. It combines periods of intense lateral thinking and generation of ideas with intense critique and ranking methods, such as the Delphi method. Guided by an iterative approach, one problem-solves by applying the tools that appear to fit best, identifies a plan, tests and improves it, and then implements it. The results will tell you whether the analytic and design process was right; if the result is an improvement, you have proven the worth of the approach you used and of the plan you developed. If not, one can refine the plan, try again, or pivot and return to the drawing board to try another tool or approach.

If the gap and your proposed intervention are too easy, you have wasted the opportunity. We urge you to take on a problem that is significant and propose a solution that is a stretch. This is a learning opportunity. We encourage you to tackle a big problem in your country with an intervention that is high impact and a challenge to carry off.

There are many ways to generate new concepts. Some of these approaches have been popularized over many years of experience. Others are our own ideas. We hope you will try some of them out and see what you think. Our suggested process of invention can be done in any sequence. There is nothing predetermined about the process we suggest. Some of the best design ideas come out of the blue.

We will roughly structure the process into the following steps: (i) establishing first impressions, in which you draw on what you have learned and experienced thus far in the study of your country; (ii) understanding and describing the problem and its root causes—understanding the problem and system gaps deeply through detailed description, and identifying the underlying causal links and root causes of the gap that your goal is intended to fix; (iii) using associative processes to broaden your understanding of the possible causes of each system gap and to benchmark ideas; (iv) exploring system components most amenable to change in the health system; (v) applying tools and ideas we have used to facilitate the creative process (but have not been rigorously evaluated); (vi) winnowing down your ideas and selecting the best; and (vii) preparing your SIP and getting ready to defend it.

Establishing First Impressions and Ideas

First impressions are an important source of innovation. You have been studying and thinking anew about your country and its problems. You may already have begun to develop ideas for change. The first step is to capture these ideas while they are still fresh.

You should first harvest ideas that have already emerged from early chapters and from the strengths and weakness, opportunities and threats (SWOT) exercise from Chapter 4 of this volume. On individual sheets of paper, you separately write your group's choice of health system's vision, your own SWOT analysis (especially opportunities and threats), and the two or three goals/gaps that the group ranked as priority problems to fix. Next, taking a broad and impressionistic view of the system and its parts, you should write down any change ideas, reactions, or thoughts that have come to mind thus far.

You can use your prior SWOT to help you generate new ideas. Figure 5.2 is a simple graphic model describing this process. Remembering your SWOT analysis and the listing of strengths and weaknesses and your responses on the spider diagram, think about how well the strengths and weaknesses align now with the goals you identified. Does this affirm your conclusion about where the system needs to improve? Then compare your identified opportunities and threats to your group's priority goals for the country. Cycling through each of your own and group's two or three selected goals for the population's health, you can look for connections between the goals and your own list of opportunities and threats. You can rank opportunities and threats from the most to least. Are there associations between where your group has tentatively decided that the country needs to be and any of the opportunities or threats? Hopefully, Step 5 will point to one of the top

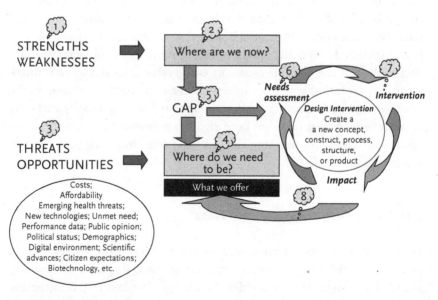

Figure 5.2 Planning roadmap.

priority gaps and goals that your group identified at the end of Chapter 4. Think about the gaps (Step 5) between where your country is and where it needs to be. Do any intervention ideas about that gap come to mind? The question is, What goal or gap is best aligned with both the system's performance and capacities (strengths and weaknesses) and its context (opportunities and threats)? What kind of intervention does that alignment make you think of? Once an intervention is identified, think about why it might work (Step 8). Write each intervention idea down, with a brief description.

Understanding and Describing the Problem and Diagnosing Its Root Causes

The field of systems theory describes a diagnostic process with four phases: (i) identifying and describing events, (ii) discerning patterns, (iii) determining if these patterns point to an underlying causal structural problem, and (iv) developing interventions. As illustrated in Figure 5.3, there are structured steps for each of these phases.

Systems communicate via expressions of their problems and successes. These include performance results, participant's complaints, surprises, and so forth. These messages are codes emanating from a health system's strains, stresses, and successes generated by the activities happening within

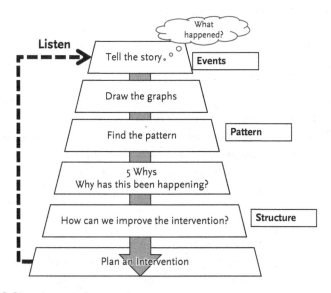

Figure 5.3 Listening to an intervention.

it. Listen to the messages and see if they could be associated with any of your selected goals and system gaps. Decoding these will help you to decipher the problem(s) underlying the gap. Proposing a diagnosis for the underlying sequence of actions may trigger a possibility for an intervention.

The first step in understanding what a system is doing is to describe its problems. There are several helpful early phase approaches or methods to characterize the problem or event.

Telling a Story

It is often useful to create a story about what you are observing. Think of yourself as a reporter and write a news article describing what you have observed and are hearing.

- Write a headline for your article.
- Begin your inquiry with the evidence. What are some of the facts that make you or others think there is an issue? Pick out the most salient features of what you are seeing and describe those.
- What happened? What's the issue? What are some of the notable events?

Charting the Trends

It is important to place the events in a context and a timeline. Do they represent a number of events that are occurring over time (and thus can show a trend)? Are there other events that involve other people or settings but may be unseen (with events being like the tip of an iceberg)? In either case, you need to act as a sleuth and determine what else is going on. Once you have described what you are observing, you are in a position to ask others if and when they are seeing similar cases or events.

The data you gather will give you a sense about (i) how frequent or common the events and problems are and (ii) what is happening over time. The latter is revealed by plotting events against a timeline.

The questions to ask are

- What's been happening?
- How have the events progressed over time?
- Have there been changes or other trends showing up over time?
- Do these changes over time begin to look like a pattern?

Doing a System Walk

Flow charting is another process that can describe and help you visualize a problem and the context in which it is occurring. One way to gather data for a flow diagram is by doing a *system walk*. For example, let's say the problem is that patients have to wait too long for an appointment. You might take a system walk in which you track all the steps from the moment a patient decides to make an appointment through to the time a clinician sees them. Using Post-its®, you write down each step or action and place them in order. You should pay special attention to steps that create a roadblock. For example, a roadblock might be created when patients must complete a form confirming insurance enrollment, which leads to a lengthy process before they can move to the next step in the process.

By placing these Post-its® in their sequence and drawing flow arrows, one can construct a map of the process flow. Once you have the flow chart in mind, you can then look for clues as to the causes of backups, factors that are wasteful and duplicative, and gaps that may create the problem that you are studying.

Looking for Patterns

Patterns may begin to emerge when you clarify the purpose of your analysis. For this reason, it is always a useful step to draft a *focusing* question or to ask the question, "What are we trying to accomplish?" For example, the following is a well-structured question: "Why, despite our improving insurance coverage, do we continue to have delays or disruptions in accessing primary care?" The patterns that emerge from your response to the question help explain the gap between the observed reality and the desired goals.

Describing and Understanding Root Causes

We will follow a well-known process for understanding the root causes of the gap you have identified and the goal you selected. This same process can be applied to all ranges of problems by posing a set of questions: What are the causes of the problem you have selected and which is the root cause— the deepest and most fundamental? What explains the patterns? Most experts suggest that conducting a root cause analysis of each of the high priority goals will help you understand why these particular gaps emerged and problems developed. Understanding their causes should help you to think up design solutions for closing the gap.

Root cause analysis (RCA) is a semi-systematic analysis of problems or events in order to understand their cause. The RCA process identifies and describes the problem clearly, creates a causal map linking the problem with its predisposing events and helps identify the most important instrumental factors from among the many that might contribute to the problem. In the course of RCA, you determine what happened, how did it happen, and why did it happen? The objective of RCA is to identify the most fundamental reason the problem emerged.

There are a number of tools commonly used to facilitate RCA. We describe the 5 Whys analysis, mind mapping, cause-and-effect diagram (the fishbone diagram), and Pareto analysis. Any or all can be of use as you conduct a root cause analysis of the gap or problem that are attempting to overcome to get to the chosen goal.

The 5 Whys Analysis

The 5 Whys is a frequently used approach in root cause analysis. The 5 Whys is a simple problem-solving technique that helps users get to the root cause of the problem quickly. It was made popular in the 1970s by the Toyota Production System. This strategy involves looking at a problem and asking "Why?" and "What caused this problem?" Often the answer to the first "why" prompts a second "why" and so on, providing the basis for the name 5 Whys.

In the 5 Whys, you select a gap, a story, a policy, or a procedure and ask "why" it is done this way. Then ask the "why" question repeatedly—five or more times, probing each answer that you get. With each "why" one digs deeper into the underlying rationale for the action. In many cases, the process reveals procedures or actions that have been inherited from earlier system designs intended to solve a problem that may no longer be present. We show (Figure 5.4) an example of the 5 Whys approach used to identify root causes of high cardiovascular disease burden in a middle-income country.

Taking your own first choice of gap or problem, conduct a root cause analysis using the 5 Whys approach to determine the most likely causes of the gap or problem. Pick the goal or problem your group selected as the most important priority for health system change or reform to address current or emerging challenges or potential opportunities. Repeat the exercise with at least one other of the gaps you selected in chapter 4.

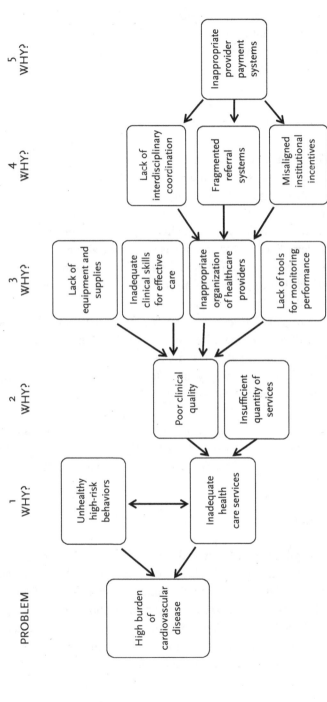

Figure 5.4 Root cause analysis of high cardiovascular disease burden.

Reversing and retracing the identified 5-why steps has the interesting property of mapping a possible intervention. Each "why" is connected to the next as one digs deeper into identifying the root cause; reversing the process and asking what it would take to get from the root cause to the next higher level of causal factors and so forth, up to the goal, creates a possible plan of intervention steps.

Mind Mapping

As discussed earlier, another approach in RCA is to brainstorm all the different elements or steps you can associate with the event or the pattern. This can be done using a technique called *mind mapping*.[1] In this technique, you write the problem in the center of a large sheet of paper and link it by lines to as many factors as you can think of that are associated in any way with the problem. Each factor and line is described with a single word, if at all possible. The brainstorming should be as free as possible, with a minimum of self-editing or deep reflection. Go for speed and flights of fancy rather than analytic rigor.

Let's say your goal is to reduce 'no-shows' at office visits to doctors. You did a system walk and generated a process flow diagram that illustrates the sequence of steps that a patient and the administrative staff take in setting up the visit. As a next step you could do a mind map. An example of a mind map for thinking about associations with first access care is shown in Figure 5.5.

The mind map is a way to make associations and link them causally. To know what to change, one needs to determine the associations that are most likely to be causal and are frequent and/or powerful effects.

Cause-and-Effect Diagram (Fishbone Diagram)

A fishbone diagram, or Ishikawa diagram, is another frequently used method in root cause analysis. Derived from the quality management process, it's an analytic tool that provides a systematic way of looking at effects and the causes that create or contribute to those effects. Because of the function of the fishbone diagram, it may be referred to as a cause-and-effect diagram. The design of the diagram looks much like the skeleton of a fish—hence the designation *fishbone* diagram.

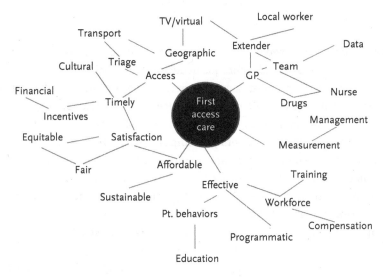

Figure 5.5 Mind map example.

This type of diagram is a line and word picture showing the most meaningful relationships between an effect and its possible causes. It is a way of graphically displaying and organizing possible causes so that it is easier to visualize possible root causes. An example of a cause and effect diagram for first access care is shown in Figure 5.6.

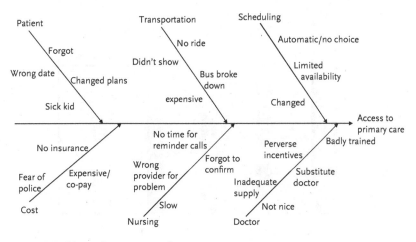

Figure 5.6 Fishbone diagram example.

Pareto analysis is used to quantify the magnitude of the cause–effect relationship—a statistical technique in decision making that is used for analysis of a selected number of tasks that produce significant overall effect. The premise is that 80% of problems are produced by a few critical causes (20%).

A Pareto chart is used to quantify factors that contribute to a problem in descending order of frequency or importance. A Pareto chart is useful in showing the most important component parts or contributors to a problem. You list contributors to a problem in order from largest to smallest or strongest to weakest. The chart then reveals the "vital few" that are contributing most to the problem.

For example, you could conduct a survey testing specific associations from a mind map. In such a survey, you might draw from a sample of patients who fail to show up for their visit. You might follow up with the staff in interviews and with each patient by phone, categorizing the cause of the no-show. Alternatively, you might ask the staff to estimate the frequency of different reasons for no shows.

The Pareto chart is a bar chart that shows the resulting frequency distribution. An example is given in Figure 5.7. The Pareto principle is a rough rule that says that about 20% of the reasons cause about 80% of the outcome.

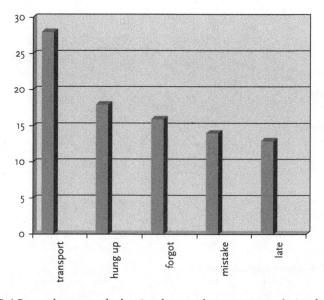

Figure 5.7 A Pareto chart example showing the most frequent causes of missed visits.

There are many other tools that can assist in RCA. We include (Box 5.3) a brief listing of other approaches commonly used in RCAs.

Box 5.3: ADDITIONAL METHODS USED IN ROOT
CAUSE ANALYSIS

- *Barrier analysis*—an investigation or design method that involves the tracing of pathways by which a target is adversely affected by a hazard, including the identification of any failed or missing countermeasures that could or should have prevented the undesired effect(s).
- *Change analysis*—looks systematically for possible risk impacts and appropriate risk management strategies in situations where change is occurring. This includes situations in which system configurations are changed, operating practices or policies are revised, new or different activities will be performed, etc.
- *Failure mode and effects analysis*—a systems engineering process that examines failures in products or processes.
- *Causal factor tree analysis*—an investigation and analysis technique used to record and display, in a logical, tree-structured hierarchy, all the actions and conditions that were necessary and sufficient for a given consequence to have occurred.
- *Fault tree analysis*—the event is placed at the root (top event) of a tree of logic. Each situation causing effect is added to the tree as a series of logic expressions.

Using Associative Processes to Broaden Understanding of the Possible Causes of the Systems Gap and to Benchmark Others' Experiences to Look for New Ideas

Most change processes benefit from generating a large list of intervention ideas. These ideas can come from any number of activities, including

- Finding out how others have addressed a similar problem. In industry, this is called *benchmarking*, and it largely occurs through informal networks of individuals. For example, if improving access is your goal, you would want to tap into the experience of experts in other countries, either through literature reports or by networking to connect with those who were involved. There may also be experts at your hospital, academic health center, consulting firms, or political staff who know something about the problem or process you plan to improve.

- Talking intensely with customers or citizens about their experiences, needs, ideas, and views can be a major source of new ideas. Many change strategies have started from those engaged in the system or the enterprise. Intense customer engagement is a key feature of one popular design methodology called *design thinking*,
- Brainstorming exercises:
  - Mind mapping. See example in Figure 5.5. Mind mapping is applicable here, as a way to structure soliciting a wide collection of intervention ideas.
  - Lateral thinking.[3] The entire book by Edward de Bono is a classic about how to think creatively. Many techniques and approaches are explained.
  - Brainstorming. Try brainstorming ideas with small groups of people who represent different groups of participants.
- Focus groups. In focus groups, participants are drawn from the system and their views gathered through a semi-structured process, which are then content analyzed.
- Site visits. Site visits to other health systems allow you to examine how they are structured and how they solve problems.
- Benchmarking. Benchmark against other country's systems from the descriptive literature or media.
- Trips to meet and talk with the participants in your or other health systems. These include businesses, insurers, providers, government, and patients.
- Loose–tight structured problem-solving. This combines periods of intense lateral thinking and generation of ideas with intense critique and ranking methods, such as the Delphi method.

Exploring in Detail System Components Most Amenable to Change in the Health System

In the model your group constructed for your country in Chapter 2 of this volume, the functions category is often expected to be the primary locus of change that policymakers can modify to improve the health system. The framework selected three functions—governance and organization, financing, and resource management—that are used to produce the system outputs (delivery of public health and personal healthcare services). You have described the status and impact of these functions on your country's health system. Therefore, you already know a great deal about how and whether these input functions are susceptible to being changed. These three functions are accessible levers that can be moved about to modify the outputs of your health system. By asking "'What if I were to change this function?" you may conjecture about new outputs that could stimulate your thinking about interventions to achieve your goal.

- Governance and organization: how functions, responsibilities, authority, and influence are distributed within your country's system. For example, we could examine the degree of decentralization, the extent of regulation, the role of competition, and the mixture of public and private sector involvement. What if the existing model were eliminated or flipped to its opposite? What might happen? Does it generate any ideas of interventions?
- Financing: the analysis should briefly consider the sources of financing (e.g., tax, insurance, out-of-pocket payments), modifying the sources of financing, how finances are pooled, whether they are allocated to agencies or intermediary organizations (such as local authorities), and how financial coverage is provided for population groups. The analysis could also briefly explore which provider payment methods are used to remunerate healthcare service providers and the pros and cons of the methods used.
- Resource management: The exercise might explore how and where financial, physical, human, and intellectual resources are allocated and whether resource shortages or distributional imbalances exist. What if resources were dramatically cut back and directed elsewhere in the system? You may also ask and conjecture what might happen to system outputs, their mix, and the way they are delivered or their distribution was altered.
- Service delivery: Public health and personal healthcare services serve overlapping but mostly distinctive health system needs. What might happen to your goal if one or the other was suddenly expanded greatly? Does the answer sound like an improvement in reaching your system goal? Is either sector able to meet current needs?

Imagine perusing the forces available to drive your change process and using them as a way to envisage what kind of influences might best energize heading to your goal. There are a number of drivers, or forces, that propel and shape a change process. We have made a tentative list of them as follows, along with our suggestion about how the output of each driver influences a process. Use this list to identify what approaches feel most appropriate to your goal and what action steps fit best with that choice of approach. This may provide clues about the sequence of steps in your causal chain.

- Hortatory, to persuade: What is the most important thing to communicate to convince people about the change needed to achieve our group's goal?
- Regulatory, to control: What would we regulate that would make a difference?
- Market forces, to compete and survive: How could the pressures of participant's preferences (consumer power) help?
- Culture/shared values to reframe beliefs and interpretations: Is there an attitude that will crop up and block the process of change? That blockage points to a causal step in your intervention.
- Management, to watch, react and adapt: Where is the most unpredictability and highest risk in moving your intervention along?

Applying Tools and Ideas We Have Used to Facilitate the Creative Process

Here are several completely speculative ideas that have seemed to work for the two of us when struggling with a knotty problem that has no known or deducible solution in sight. The first is the advice to loosen up. Doodle, draw incomplete diagrams, google for any associations, and let yourself be completely immersed in the problem without forcing a solution.

The second is to find a "victim" to talk with about the problem—or even better, to debate with. Try to outline the problem, what you think is causing it, and any thoughts about how to fix it. We have found that good ideas often pop up in the course of attempting to make an argument in a discussion or debate.

The third thing that has worked for us is to use early morning for what we imagine might be right brain functioning (i.e., the nonlogical side of the brain). Go to bed thinking about the problem. Wake up an hour or two before your usual time but stay in or go back to bed. If you know how to meditate, do so. If not, just lie quietly letting your mind wander. Let associations come and go. Keep a pad of paper nearby to write down any ideas that occur to you. This has been a particularly fruitful time for problem-solving for us.

The final piece of advice is to write a description of ideas regardless of how good you think they are and put them out of sight until a later review after a few days. It is always sobering to see how bad the writing is but also to have fresh insight into fixing the problem.

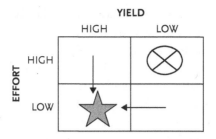

Figure 5.8 Mapping yield against effort of a proposed intervention.

Winnowing Down Your Ideas

Once you are satisfied that you have generated some good interventions, it is time to narrow them down to no more than one or two that you will present at your country group meeting. To start this process, you should make a list of your intervention ideas and display them next to your group's priority problem. Of course, it may be immediately clear which of these is the best. Great! But, even so, we suggest two activities that will confirm your choice or, if you are unsure, may help you focus your SIP. These are, first, evaluating each candidate against a yield/effort 2 × 2 table, and, second, assessing your top options by beginning to prepare your formal SIP.

Conduct a benefit/effort exercise for each proposed intervention step. Take your list of intervention options and assign them to the appropriate spot on the 2 × 2 yield/effort table (Figure 5.8). Try to improve your ideas in the direction of the star quadrant. Those that are easy but low yield may require some further thinking to determine if they can be made more impactful. Other ideas in the high-yield and high-effort quadrant are definitely worth thinking about more. Their implementation effort might be lessened with further reflection or if broken up into feasible phases. See if you can move ideas in either of the two quadrants into the star category. Discard those that fall into the high-effort, low-yield quadrant, unless you have a breakthrough in imagining how you could improve its score.

Preparing Your System Improvement Plan and Getting Ready to Defend It

The last step in your homework assignment is to produce your draft SIP following the outline (Box 5.2). Your SIP should be a two-page (maximum) description of your target problem and a detailed explanation of the potential intervention(s) that you are considering. This plan should be transmitted to the colleagues with whom you are working in your small subgroup.

Be rigorous in self-assessing your SIP. You want to explain your thinking in some detail, to give specifics about your assumptions, and to defend your logic. Testing yourself for the strength of your explanations and justifications is key. Spend time exploring your explanations of the connections between the gaps and goals, problem formulation and its root causes, and your proposed connecting causative steps in the intervention. You should be able to convince yourself that the causal linkages in the sequence of steps of the intervention are real and strong. If they aren't, your work hasn't really been completed.

Don't accept a facile or superficial plan from yourself. Like a good application for research funding, your selected problem should be significant. Its solution should make a difference in the targeted results for your health system. Your intervention should be rigorous—high impact but feasible to implement. Your probing and challenging at this semi-final design stage will make a difference in what you learn and in whether your ideas might be selected to be implemented. Don't make this too easy for yourself. It's better to go back for another round of thinking, observation, interviews, and data collection than to give an answer that you are not happy with.

Finishing the Group's Systems Improvement Plan

Small Group Meeting

Use a second small group meeting to reach a conclusion and finalize the SIP for the group. Your independent work is complete; you have taken the feedback from your colleagues, made revisions, finished your SIP, and readied it for presentation at the meeting of your country group. You will have written up your plan according to the format in Box 5.2. Upon arrival at the meeting, each will have prepared their SIP and arranged to be first reviewer of another student's plan and second reviewer of the remaining proposal. First reviewers are expected to evaluate the SIP in depth and to provide actionable feedback to the proposer.

At your second and final country group meeting, each member will present their revised and improved SIP. The group will discuss and critique each SIP proposal's strengths and weaknesses. The group will decide which SIP, or combination thereof, the group should select and prepare for implementation. Activities in this group process will include discussion of impact, cost, and feasibility using the yield/effort table, trading off of ideas among students, and designing their final group SIP. The group will write up their SIP in preparation for the next chapter—the test and improve stage.

Optional All Groups Meeting

If there is time, the program director should schedule a final meeting of all the groups to present and discuss each small group's proposed SIP. The presentation should be brief, covering their vision, gaps, and goals; proposed intervention (displayed as a causal chain); their proposed outcome and impact on the goals; and the rationale for their approach. Each presentation will be followed by questions and suggestions.

CHAPTER 6

Testing the Change, Improving the Plan

Ever tried? Ever failed? No matter. Try again. Fail again. Fail better.
—Samuel Beckett

INTRODUCTION

The goal of this chapter is to test, refine, and prepare each student's system improvement plan (SIP) for implementation. Participants will revisit their country SIP to tune its constituent process steps. They will produce a process flow map of their plan starting with its inputs, building the change through sequential action steps and ultimately producing the outputs that enable the SIP to attain its goals.

Then they will conduct one or more test runs to improve their SIP and increase their confidence that it will deliver the outputs they need. It is hard to predict the results of change in a complex dynamic system with much hope of getting it right the first time. For this reason, most plans are best subjected to iterative cycles of testing. For this we introduce a process called a *model for improvement* that helps designers test and improve their plan. Using this model, participants will test their intervention, progressively strengthen its design, and prepare it for implementation. With each cycle of testing, the designer gains confidence that the plan will work.

We introduce the topic of measuring results. We will discuss how the initiator of a plan, from a policy person or a chief executive to a parliament or an executive body, can assess if it has been successful or not. The process of assessment involves setting and measuring goals and targets. We discuss the challenges of measurement in healthcare where much that is important is not obviously or easily measurable and where finding metrics and measures of success is a challenge.

Finally, we present a systems framework to make an informed decision about implementation. Whether the change agent is a presenter of a plan or its funder and sponsor, they need a way to decide how best to move forward with a proposed system change plan. Using this framework, the participants will assess their own and others' SIPs to understand their potential impact, effort, feasibility, and risks. They will understand what type of development their SIP will need, who will implement it, and how.

THE STUDENT WORK PLAN

Your objectives for this chapter are to learn how to test, critique, refine, improve, and decide when and whether to implement your SIP. You will work on your own SIP from Chapter 5 of this volume to improve its conception and construction. You will apply the model for improvement to move your SIP through a virtual test run of improvement. In this full-cycle test, you determine the measures of success, assess the results, and diagnose what causes problems or creates opportunities for improvement.

Each of you will work twice on your own, with each round of independent work followed by a meeting in your country-specific subgroups. You will first be introduced to our own version of W. Edwards Deming's historical plan–do–study–act (PDSA) for improvement, a trial and error, data-based feedback system developed in the 1950s for automobile manufacturing in Japan. We call our version the D3A3 model. Using the D3A3 model, individuals will develop measures of success on their own and then propose to the group their thoughts about how to measure results in each step of the plan. In the first round, each student in your group will independently develop and then present to the group their version of the country SIP intervention process, breaking the process into manageable pieces, describing the sequential steps of the plan, and specifying its proposed output and outcomes. You will portray your plan in the form of a flow diagram over time (called a program evaluation review technique [PERT] chart), showing the critical implementation pathway from its beginning to the proposed end result. The small group will discuss and agree on one version of the plan to work on in the second round. Once your student group has agreed on a uniform plan, each student will pick one of the process steps for further development and improvement in a second round of self-study.

During the second round of independent study, each of you will practice using the D3A3 model as though you were conducting a test both of your assigned sub element and the group's overall planned SIP. You will apply the D3A3 improvement framework through one complete round of virtual testing, examining the likely achievement of results and predicting the reactions of those stakeholder groups that would be affected by the change. Each student will prepare a summary of what the implementers of their SIP will have to do to make the change work.

The small groups will meet a second time for critique, feedback, and discussion. Each student will propose an implementation map, summarizing the results of their testing and improvement thru the D3A3 cycle. After brief presentations of the improvement process and proposed steps, the group will discuss and agree on a unified SIP plan to reach their change goal, comprising their agreed sequence of steps and D3A3 tests. The group will plan their SIP's implementation proposal and design a storyboard to be presented at this chapter's wrap-up large group meeting.

In the final step of this chapter, all country groups will meet to present their plan for their SIP and to critique each other's proposals.

GENERAL APPROACH TO TESTING FOR IMPLEMENTATION

Implementing change in any system, even when the planner is fortunate enough to be planning a green field health system, is filled with uncertainty. Predicting exactly how a system will respond to a change in design is extremely difficult. Health systems exhibit dynamic complexity. They are homeostatic; they resist change. Understanding the system is critically important, since any change generates consequences as the system fights back. The greater the difference between the current system's processes and its predicted successor, the greater the uncertainty and risk.

A robust plan should make us confident that it will produce the predicted improvement. The stronger the planner's confidence in their capacity to predict the results of each action, the greater the certainty that the planned outcome will actually deliver what is planned. The certainty that a plan will achieve the results we want is dependent on the strength of our belief in that prediction. If our belief is based on repeated evidence of success in similar circumstances, our confidence in achieving the desired result is great. If untested, the risk of failure or the possibility of unintended consequences is elevated.

One's confidence is based on an underlying explanatory causal model that is supposed to make it possible to predict the results of a change. The certainty of a plan's prediction is only as good as the reliability and prognostic strength of the assumptions built into its causal model or mechanisms. The more that is known, the more reliable are the predictions of the outputs and the greater the confidence that carrying out the plan will lead to the proposed goal. When knowledge is strong and scientifically tested, the designer can predict the results and impact with accuracy and knows what and how to measure. For example, a lot is known about how gasoline ignites in the cylinder of a combustion motor. Designing a modification in its structure leading to a change in its performance can be predicted with some confidence. On the other hand, changing a payment model for doctors deals with a multitude of interacting and sometimes conflicting goals, values, responsibilities (in both public and private sectors), and the reactions of others such as patients and payers. Less is known about the actions in the plan and the predictability of producing the required result is uncertain.

To reduce the uncertainty of a proposed change, the approach most prevalent today is twofold: first, break the plan up into steps and, second, test and improve each step before implementing. The first activity in this approach is to make a plan that deconstructs the overall system change into bite-sized chunks. Each chunk corresponds to a step in a pathway leading from the *status quo* towards the new outcomes. Usually, each step's successful output becomes the input to the next, in a sequence ultimately producing the proposed outcome.

To increase predictability that a plan will achieve its intended results, we run what amount to tests. Trial runs are undertaken before implementing a full change process, such as your proposed SIP. The operational objective of the test cycle is to determine whether a change happened and if that change led to an improvement. A rigorous method of inquiry facilitates learning from the testing experiences.

The purpose of trial runs using the D3A3 framework is to improve the elements, overall plan, and design of a system change to reduce risk and uncertainty inherent in working in complex, dynamic systems. Improvement cycles are the planner's opportunity to predict the likelihood of success, reduce the risks of change, and modify the design to improve the results.

Testing and improving each step increases one's confidence in the success of the plan when finally implemented. Each run is an experiment; as the test results emerge, learning occurs. Progress is made through testing, learning, and improvement from repeating improvement cycles on critical steps in the change process pathway.

The D3A3 Model

The D3A3 model for improvement is our adaptation of the PDSA cycle to guide testing, assessing, and improving an SIP in a health system. In our

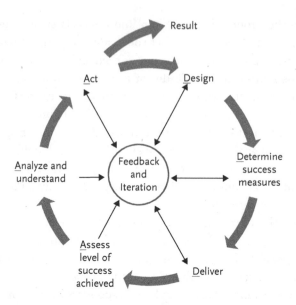

Figure 6.1 D3A3 model for improvement diagram.

D3A3 modification of the PDSA approach, each of the now six stages is a sequential step in the change process (Figure 6.1). The flow is progressive: from designing the change to determining the results you expect and will measure to carrying out the change, assessing what happened, analyzing and interpreting the results and adapting the design plan so as to improve its performance the next time through. At the beginning of each new improvement cycle, the designer resets the measures of success and assesses how well the remedial efforts have worked.

The D3A3 process is applied to each step in the causal chain leading to the desired result. Successful implementation nudges the system in steps through a linked succession of new states that are iteratively developed, each vectoring toward the eventual planned system goal. Signals may emanate from any of the steps as the process proceeds, so feedback, ongoing learning, and iteration can be both opportunistic and continuous. This process is shown graphically in Figure 6.2, which shows the D3A3 framework superimposed on each of the linked sequential steps of a total change process.

Each step can be tested, evaluated, adjusted, and improved until its output is optimized and the prediction of its success is strong enough to proceed to implementation. At the point where the learning plateaus, the process advances to the next step until all steps have been piloted and

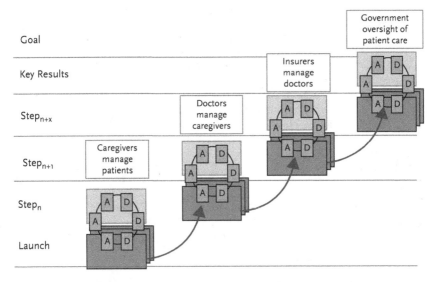

Figure 6.2 Example of sequential D3A3 test cycles applied to care oversight.

improved. The planner has then done what they can to test the change and is ready to implement—or abandon—the plan. When the improvement loop ceases to stimulate improvements, the cycling stops, and the last result is accepted as the final output of that process. That output is the input to the next step in the overall change process.

First Independent Study: Applying the D3A3 Improvement Cycle to Your SIP

The learning activity for this chapter is to apply the D3A3 improvement model to your SIP.

The first step is to apply the D3A3 model design to at least one, or more, of your project plan's implementation steps in the causal chain. These steps are the pathway of actions (like stepping stones). Applying the D3A3 model tests the sequencing, interrelationships, and interdependencies of each stage that will be followed as the plan moves into action. Working on your own now, your activity before your initial country group meeting is to complete the three Ds in the model for improvement.

Keep track of your progress using the D3A3 process. As you run through the D3A3 model's six steps, summarize your findings in Table 6.1.

The steps in the D3A3 assignment are as follows.

Table 6.1 SUMMARY OF THE D3A3 CYCLE ON A SELECTED CAUSAL CHAIN STEP

Describe the Target Step(s) in the Causal Chain

Stage in D2A2 Model	Describe and List Features	Results from Trial Run	Reactions, Responses, and Notes
D1: Design the intervention plan			
D2: Determine the measures of success			
D3: Deliver			
A1: Assess			
A2: Analyze			
A3: Act			

D1: Design the Intervention Plan

In the D1 activity of applying the improvement model, you will describe in detail the steps in the planned intervention to which you are applying the D3A3 cycle. At the end of Chapter 5 of this volume, each country group identified a gap, picked a goal, and proposed an SIP change plan. The D1 process builds upon that product of the prior chapter. Return to your SIP now to do a high-level update of your plan. First, you will reaffirm your plan's appropriateness and feasibility. You will review the construction of your group's change process. You will revisit the steps in the causal chain through which you will deliver your intended result, adding detail to it and confirming that the output of each step is an input to the next and that the sequence of steps is the most efficient, effective, and feasible way to move from initiating the change to producing its desired results. The questions to ask include "What problem(s) are we trying to solve?" "What are we trying to accomplish?" "What change output and outcome has to happen at each step to move the change process along?" and "How confident am I that these action steps will deliver the result we need"?

We suggest several tools to facilitate this process: flow charts; a SMART determination of measurable outcomes (which we describe in detail later); and the yield/effort matrix, which was introduced in Chapter 5 of this volume. Although highlighted in this chapter, these three tools are useful in almost all steps of conceptualizing, constructing, and implementing a system change.

Your initial assignment is to create a time-sequenced flow chart of your SIP, showing the optimal path to the end result. You display this path by representing your overall SIP plan in the form of a PERT chart, an advanced version of a flow diagram that was developed by the US navy in the 1950s. A PERT chart organizes a multistep project in steps against a time line, interconnects the steps, and arranges their timing according to the sequence through which the project must proceed. From these relationships, one can calculate the critical pathway from beginning to end; the shorter the time line is, the more efficient the project. See how far you can get in transforming your causal chain flow diagram into a PERT/critical path chart as illustrated generically in Figure 6.3.

A PERT chart is not the only way to communicate the design of your SIP. Various other forms of flow charts could be useful at this stage of implementation. These range from simple steps in a time sequence to sophisticated charting representing the process symbolically with special shapes (rectangles, ovals, etc.) indicating structure, sequence, and relationships.

Another useful process tool is represented by the acronym SMART. SMART is a tool developed for management[1] and expanded for use in patients planning a personal change in a health behavior such as smoking or obesity. SMART stands for specific, measurable, achievable, relevant, and time-bound. This checklist emphasizes the criteria needed to achieve measurable results that are a stretch but still feasible. You can use the SMART questions to ask yourself if each step in your SIP's causal chain is meaningful and achievable with a reasonable effort by those participating in the actions. Finally, SMART reminds us that operating within time limits is a practical necessity, a motivator, and an important measure of performance.

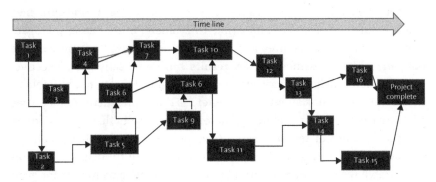

Figure 6.3 PERT chart example.

The third tool assesses the value of each step in the SIP sequence. A yield/effort matrix is a 2 × 2 table of effort (see Figure 5.8 in Chapter 5), where yield is thought of as the outcome that is the best input to the next step in the sequence. One assigns each implementation step to a quartile of the yield/effort table and thinks, impressionistically, about how to redesign the step to lower the effort and enhance impact. The framework makes it possible to estimate how hard each step will be to carry out and whether one can increase its benefit/cost.

D2: Determine the Measures of Success

The designer's first step in assessing a plan for change is to predict the result as best they can and strive to select measures likely to inform an observer if the actual outcome was the result that was expected. In this step, you will define measures to evaluate whether the trial run has attained the outputs you sought from your design. Observing what happens as a result of testing your plan is of critical importance to improvement. What gets evaluated drives performance. What gets measured gets done. Without assessment of performance there is no way to know if your intervention has worked. Ask yourself, "What are the measures of success at each step? How will I know that my plan has generated the planned outputs or results"?

It is important to clarify and define your measures of success in advance. Measurement is an imperfect science. The meaning of important performance terms like *quality*, *satisfaction*, and *wellness* are often vague and interpreted differently among people. Multiple parties participate in the design of measurement systems and are influenced by planned change. Their reactions often differ, sometimes in ways that bias results. The clearer one can be about what one is measuring, the more that one can learn from the trial run.

There are many ways to measure success or failure. Measuring outcomes is ideal, but they often are impossible to evaluate; in that case, surrogate measures such as structures and processes can be used to approximate outcomes. The assessment of key results can be objective or subjective, with the latter including attitudes, emotions, and feelings, quantifiable or not. One way to think about measurement is that while there are measures that you can predict and quantify, there are also results that you can know and predict but not measure easily (e.g., people's mood, beliefs, feelings, and attitudes). In this section, you should take care to focus not just on measurable results, but also carefully consider what signs to look for even though formal measurement might not be feasible.

There are also outcomes that you neither know nor can predict. In this latter category are surprises, errors, unexplained variation, complaints, logjams, and conflicts; one rarely knows their root causes in advance (remember the dynamic complexity of health systems and unintended consequences of actions). Listening for and interpreting these unpredicted events is vitally important for improving design structures and processes, especially those that are complicated.

If a quantitative representation of the output or outcome is possible, the planner should use it. Statistical methods and tests can be used when it is important to determine if the change represents chance variation and to assess just how significant the change is. The determination of significance ranges from the most simple impressions of expected versus actual results to formal designs such as before–after comparisons, time-series, statistical process control, and factorial analysis.

In this educational exercise, you should describe one or two measures of the results—outputs, outcomes, or goals—you hope to produce from your SIP. These results can be described in either quantitative or subjective terms, and they can relate to health system inputs (functions), outputs, and outcomes (as described in our health systems framework; Figure 6.4).

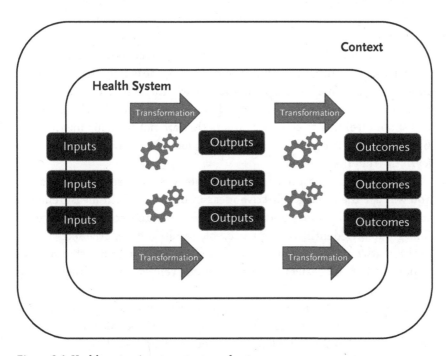

Figure 6.4 Health system inputs, outputs, and outcomes.

If it is possible, the planner should attempt to measure the end result, outcomes, or goals. For example, revisiting the descriptive system model in Chapter 2, we recall that the health system's outcomes include health, collective cost, personal financial protection, and user satisfaction. Policy interventions could aim to improve both the level and distribution of any or all of these outcomes.

Falling short of outcomes, stand-in process measures highly associated with outcomes may suffice. For example, some policies aim to improve healthcare delivery system outputs. In the Chapter 2 descriptive model, these are health services at an individual level or public health measures at a population level that planners believe are likely to improve health system outcomes. The intervention might propose to improve their equity, effectiveness, efficiency, and responsiveness.

Alternatively, policy objectives may strive to modify or improve the functions that affect health system outputs. The objectives might, for example, seek to improve or modify organizational design and governance (e.g., more or less decentralization of decision-making), financing (e.g., introducing performance related payment of healthcare providers), or resource management (such as establishing a priority-setting process or modifying an existing one; task-shifting to enable provision of healthcare services by different health workers; team-working; or enhancing supply chain management to prevent stock shortages of medicines or health products).

Table 6.2 provides some examples of health system outcomes, outputs, objectives, and functions and their related measures that could be considered to define targets or to evaluate whether a policy or change has led to any improvement (or unintended consequences). For this exercise, you should feel free to consider targets that are not formally measurable. Even just describing the results you are looking for will facilitate your learning from the test run.

As you think of measurements of your intervention steps, fill in Table 6.3. You will use the group's collective ideas in deciding which measurements to use for the outcomes and proxies (processes and structures) of your final group SIP. Identify both quantifiable results (efficiency, effectiveness, health status, patient satisfaction on surveys, etc.) and ones that may be important but not easily measured (responsiveness, equity, financial risk protection, etc.).

Knowing how much design and data collection effort to expend on a process step is an important skill. It is easy to go overboard and suffer analysis paralysis. On the other hand, it is equally dangerous to gloss over the data collection and analysis steps. They require a lot of thought and effort.

Table 6.2 EXAMPLES OF INDICATORS TO MEASURE HEALTH SYSTEM OUTCOMES, OUTPUTS, AND PROCESS FUNCTIONS

Health system outcomes	
Health	Mortality (from a condition)
	Years of life
	Disability-adjusted life years
	Well-being and happiness
	Work and family functional capacity
Financial protection	Levels of out-of-pocket expenditures as a percentage of total health spending
	Levels of catastrophic or impoverishing health expenditures (by income quintile)
User satisfaction	Measures in relation to autonomy, choice, communication, confidentiality
Economic sustainability	Healthcare expenditures as a percentage of gross domestic product
	Annual real growth rate of national healthcare expenditures
	National budget deficit
	National debt as a percentage of gross domestic product
Health system outputs	
Public health services	Proportion of interventions that use risk stratification and are targeted interventions
Individual health services	Proportion of healthcare services provided at primary healthcare setting
	Waiting times to see a clinician
Health system objectives	
Equity	Health care coverage (by socioeconomic group)
	Access to effective healthcare services (by socioeconomic group)
	Unmet need (by socioeconomic group)
Effectiveness	Per capita rates of cost-effective interventions (e.g., lipid-lowering medicines)
	Level of unwarranted interventions (e.g., Caesarean sections; antibiotic use)
	Proportion of patients receiving correct intervention or achieving effective control
	Death rates in hospital or post discharge (30 days) for specific conditions (e.g., myocardial infarction)

(continued)

Table 6.2 CONTINUED

Efficiency	Proportion of funding allocated to domains (primary healthcare vs. public health vs. hospital) Proportion of funding allocated to cost-effective interventions Average length of hospital stays (general, acute admissions, for specific conditions)
Responsiveness	Measures related to wait time; respectful communication by healthcare providers; cleanliness of the healthcare facility; freedom to choose a healthcare provider
Health system functions (inputs)	
Organization and governance	Extent of citizen involvement in policy development Centralized versus distributed (subsidiarity) authority
Financing	Use of performance-related payment systems Proportion of funding allocated to different population groups
Resource management	Use of transparent priority setting in resource allocation Proportion of expenditure on administrative functions

Table 6.3 MEASUREMENT WORKSHEET FORMAT

	Brief description of desired result(s)	Outcome measures	Surrogate measures	Results
SIP Outcome	1. 2. 3.			
Step 1 in the causal chain				
Step 2				
Step *n*				

Consider that if the process step is one with low-impact and risk, assessment can be simple and quick. If the step is critical in the change pathway or represents a high risk to the full enterprise, significant effort and a long study time can be appropriate.

Whether an outcome or its proxy can be formulated or not, the planner can identify other salient signs or symptoms to anticipate and look for. Among the most important are the initial responses of groups likely to be affected by your SIP. It is possible to make useful generalizations that enable a change agent to look for early signs of what is happening. You should be able to predict the most likely reaction to the change process in each. The questions to answer are, "Who is involved in the intervention?" "Who are the individuals and to what groups do they belong?" and "What kinds of reactions would I expect from them?"

As your next step, predict and begin to describe the responses of participants affected by your SIP, and ask yourself how they might differ in their outcomes and reactions. As a first step, make a list of the parties who will be touched by changes in the SIP plan you are proposing. Write them in Table 6.4 and specify, to the best of your ability, what you predict their general reactions would be to your change plan. With which groups do you

Table 6.4 PARTICIPANTS WHO WILL BE AFFECTED IN SOME WAY BY THE CHANGE PLAN

Participants	Predicted Reactions	Reason Why
Patients		
PCPs/GPs		
Specialists/ hospitals		
Political leaders		
Citizens		
Payers/insurers		
Other		

Abbreviations: GP, general practitioner; PCP, primary care physician.

postulate you will see the most facilitating responses or greatest barriers to change? What do you predict will be their positions and reactions to the change? Which among these participant groups is most important to a successful outcome? Imagine what they do in response to your SIP and what actions involve them. Who are likely to be the most negative and the most powerful blockers? List the reasons. What do you expect to see happen in each group as your plan is implemented? What problems would you predict as a result? Pick the most likely to resist and go back and make sure that you have measures for early mitigation.

Also make an informed guess about what might be happening but is not predictable. What might you hear or see if you were watching carefully for unknown events? Think about how to create sensors or listening processes that would enable you to hear about this type of feedback from the process. Understanding whether these are forming a pattern and to what underlying design issue they might be reacting is important, especially in systems dynamics modeling and looking for classic archetypal design issues. A good place to look is for delays or waiting times.

D3: Deliver

Imagine carrying out the trial run. Visualize the experience by walking the critical path and visualizing the likely outcome at each step. Imagine what happens as the process plays out. Think especially about the key groups. Listen hard. Imagine what participants might say out loud or what they might be thinking. Speculate about the underlying reason for their predicted response. You should be thinking about the following perspectives: "Where am I most likely to hear early signs of resistance or enthusiasm? Are there leading indicators of either success or trouble brewing?" A leading indicator is one that shows up very early and has high sensitivity (i.e., its sensing is very easily triggered, even though a positive result is less likely to be a true case than those detected by a less sensitive indicator).

First Small Group Meeting (Two Hours)

The purpose of this session is to review progress and decide next steps. The desired outcome is for the group to coalesce around the final SIP on which all the small group members will work. The group should agree to one plan for delivering their final SIP, a commonly agreed goal, targeted output and outcomes, and a set of measures to be collecting or observing.

Participants will present, discuss, react, refine, and agree to each of the causal chain building block steps in the group's proposed SIP. Each participant will present their plan and proposed measures of success for each step. The group will discuss and suggest improvements. As the final action in this session, the group should divide up the steps in the SIP sequence among its members as their assignment for the next round so that all steps are covered.

Second Individual Study: Completing the D3A3 Model and Choosing a Plan of Action

This assignment kicks off the second round of individual study focusing on the group's single SIP. Assume that you have run the first half of the D3A3 test of the change. Return to Table 6.1 and update it with what you have learned in your small group discussion. Each student then completes the A steps in the D3A3 model for their chosen step(s), proposes an action, and prepares to present their results at the next small group meeting.

A1: Assess

You have completed The D3A3 improvement cycle virtual trial run through the delivery phase, and the study questions now are "How did it go?" "What happened?" "What were the results?" "What events did I hear about?" "Were expected results achieved, both objective and subjective?" and "Were there deviations, surprises, errors, work-arounds, etc.?"

Return to Table 6.3 to record your results for the objective and subjective measures of success you identified. Enter some likely results from your virtual test run for each of your designated evaluation measures. Where there are objective measures, they should be noted and what you observed (virtually) should be compared to expected results.

Your virtual improvement trial would have elicited reactions from the stakeholder groups. In the D2 section on determining measures of success, you speculated about behavioral responses among differing groups that would be affected by your SIP or one of its steps. Invent some believable feedback based on your predictions.

Repeat the process by conjecturing about unexpected signals from the pilot. What errors, surprises, and gaps do you imagine seeing? Box 6.1 shows some of the types of reactions that might have been observed during the test cycle. Select those you might worry the most about. In A2, we will contemplate why such responses might have occurred.

A2: Analyze and Understand

Students will study the virtual trial run results observed during the prior A1 stage, determine their root causes, and begin thinking about potential fixes. The operating question here is, "What accounts for or explains the findings?" For behavioral observations or interpersonal conflicts, the question might be "What needs to be true for these individuals for them to be behaving this way?"

The purpose of collecting this feedback from the system undergoing modification is to learn something about the system's behavior during change that points us toward a diagnosis of the cause and leads to actions for improvement. The analysis step (A2) is where you attempt to formulate a diagnosis (create and describe an explanatory model) that elucidates what you have observed during and at the end of the test run of the D3A3 model for improvement.

Generating a diagnosis is a kind of detective process. You now have a collection of data-based observations, subjective assessments, human reactions, and random nonclassifiable events. Your job is to examine the evidence (signs, symptoms, events, patterns, and variation), deduce and hypothesize mechanisms, and then test their validity. Validity is ultimately assessed by how well the diagnosis generated by the explanatory model accounts for the mechanisms creating the signals (actual outputs compared to expectations, signs and symptoms, and events and patterns emanating from the delivery of the change) and whether treatment improves the results. No hypothesis is ultimately of value unless it can be validated by demonstrating that an action based on the hypothesis actually leads to improvement.

Pick some problems from the results column in Table 6.3. Select several of these hypothetical results and see if you can develop theories about what might account for them. What could explain what went wrong? Make a list of potential diagnoses. In the act stage of the D3A3 cycle, we will work with a few of these high impact performance shortfalls and attempt to identify mitigating interventions that might fix the problems and improve performance in subsequent D3A3 cycles.

Feedback about stakeholder groups can reveal the need and target for another D3A3 improvement cycle. Imagine that you have worrisome feedback from one or more of the groups affected by implementing your SIP plan. Pick one or two as a target for improvement. Use the 5 Whys to understand the root cause of this response to change and speculate about what you might adjust to manage the resistance or reaction.

Finally, we urge you to think about the category of unpredicted events that occur recurrently but don't establish themselves into a pattern. The signals are clues that need to be incorporated into a hypothesis—a theme. The observer formulates explanatory stories to make sense of the events, looking for patterns that point to the tale being told. These events are a system's attempt to give feedback to the designer that there is a hidden problem. The challenge is to interpret what these events are communicating about the system archetype and problem. Figure 6.5 (shown first in Chapter 5 as Figure 5.3) is a variant of a root cause exercise and shows one process to follow in understanding such events.

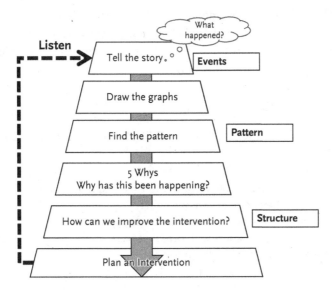

Figure 6.5 Listening to an intervention.

The traditional root cause analysis also can be helpful, as summarized in Box 6.2. Remember that the 5 Whys route to the root cause is also a roadmap to fix it when put into reverse. Each *why* answer is contributing in sequence to the final root cause of the problem you have detected. Therefore, you can run it in the opposite direction and work backwards, asking yourself what specific action steps might fix the *why* problem just preceding the final root cause and so forth in reverse order. This may be useful as you invent what to do in the final act step in the improvement cycle.

Box 6.2: ROOT CAUSE ANALYSIS—THE THINKING PROCESS

- Ask as many *whys* as necessary to identify the root cause.
- Each problem is likely to be caused by multiple, interconnected causes—identify the linkages.
- Look for actionable causes:
- Do not jump to conclusions.
- Be specific. Consider evidence to check your initial ideas.
- Root cause analysis provides the path to solutions; however, there is no one right answer.
- Work forward to identify solutions to the root causes of the problem.

The final step of Analysis is to formulate possible interventions to fix the problems your Improvement Cycle has revealed. Many of the tools of analysis and rules of the road can help in this process. Don't be discouraged with your answers. Identifying an underlying performance problem may not lead to a clean answer (Box 6.3).

Box 6.3: UNCOVERING THE PROCESS—WHAT WILL YOU DISCOVER?

Most performance problems have multiple and interconnected causes. Many causes have more than one effect.
Remember you are dealing with a complex system.
Improving performance will often require more than one action; sequencing is of critical importance.

A3: Act to Improve the Design and Decide Next Steps

The final step in each improvement cycle is to decide what actions to undertake next. The planner faces a handful of choices: such as, run more D3A3 improvement cycles for this step, move on to run improvement cycles in other steps, or proceed to full implementation of the SIP.

In this section, you will first examine the results from your D3A3 trial run and assess whether or not the step poses a risk to your intervention (or to your goals) and needs to be improved. If not, you will then decide whether to implement or not. Presenting your steps, the problems encountered, your proposed remedial solution, and the suggested action will be the basis of the second small group meeting.

Your first action in the act (A3) stage of the improvement model cycle is to take the feedback from the virtual trial run of your change project and consider if you still need to improve your plan. Review your record of results of each of the D3A3 stages from Table 6.1. Perhaps you will conclude that changes are needed in your plan and more D3A3 test cycles are required to determine if these actions will improve the results. Or, you may conclude that the improvements give you enough confidence to proceed.

Next, you will decide what changes you would make. In the analyze (A2) stage of the cycle, you used performance feedback information to develop a working understanding of the strengths and weaknesses of your SIP and its constituent causal steps. With this tentative diagnosis in hand, decide what needs to be fixed. From Table 6.2, pick one or two of the most troubling problems you encountered in the test cycle. You should identify and describe the improvements you would like to make to ameliorate these problems. Given your analysis and diagnosis of the root causes, propose modifications to improve your plan. Describe the changes and test your reasoning by asking yourself why you think this alteration will improve the result.

Your next decision is whether the changes you propose are worth the effort. You need to affirm that the improvements justify the cost, effort, and risk of the change process itself. To make this decision, the designer first must decide what more needs to be done and, when confident about the intervention, must ask what value is produced by the change—the benefit–cost. This entails making a decision based on the impact, effort, and risk of the change. This process is facilitated by returning to the yield/effort table (Figure 6.6) adding the further variable of risk. In this process, you should consider the following: can you improve the results, can you reduce the risks, can you make the step more efficient (reducing time and/or costs).

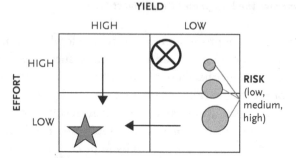

Figure 6.6 Is it worth it? Setting priorities.

Based on the feedback from your D3A3 cycle, ask yourself how much impact to expect. The first question is, how confident are you that there will be a change from your SIP? Next, will the change be an improvement? Finally, the planner answers the "So what? Who cares?" question. Is the impact important, significant, and unique? How positively will the intended beneficiaries view the change? Give the overall SIP a score for impact—small, medium, or large. You should also assess the impact of each step in advancing the change. Is it critical or not? Is it worth it to undertake interventions that will improve your plan?

Next, you should estimate the effort needed both for the individual steps and overall SIP. In balancing yield against effort, you are assessing overall impact from your SIP against the sum of effort of all the subsidiary steps.

Moreover, there is misspent effort. These are choices that are lost as the consequence of moving ahead. These are called *opportunity costs*. They include other targets or goals that your SIP will displace because it draws down shared resources. Some of these goals may be outside healthcare—education, infrastructure, or defense, if one is looking at a proposed change at a national level. Or, they may be trade-offs within healthcare, such as other healthcare service initiatives that compete with your SIP for investment.

You will want to ask if the effort matches the magnitude of the opportunity that is possible given the environmental conditions. Is there a crisis? It would be a shame to waste the momentum on a trivial change. Is there an alignment of interests? Does your proposed SIP take advantage of reinforcing alignments? Here a force field analysis might provide clues. There might be a significant stakeholder looking for big change; examples might be a new government wanting to accomplish something big or a once-in-a-lifetime charismatic leader.

The third element in your analysis is the level of risk the intervention confronts. All projects face failure and unintended consequences. Your improvement cycle was undertaken to reduce the likelihood of such events. Nevertheless, if your intervention puts an important organization or group of people at heightened risk, the impact of the change needs to be very high to warrant moving ahead. High-risk, high-effort, high-gain system changes can be worth doing, but it is important to have considered the consequences. Incorporate your estimate of the risks from failure or unintended second order consequences. Ask yourself, "What could go wrong?" and estimate how damaging that would be. Are you prepared for it, and can the risk be cushioned or eliminated? Avoid taking a big risk for a small gain.

Finally, remember that not all change is an improvement. The outputs from modifications in the system may change, whether from planned interventions from within or from unrelated shifts in the environment of the system, but these changes may not improve the outcomes. Before implementation, the designer should once again determine that the expected change leads to an improvement in the outputs and an enhanced likelihood of achieving objectives and goals of the system.

The decision about what action to undertake as you complete the D3A3 improvement cycle depends on your assessment of the step in the causal chain. You must decide whether the step is ready for implementation or needs improvement and more trial run cycles to test it. Some problems can be very complicated to fix, but if the step is critical to the success of an important SIP change, the manager of the process must intervene, test again, and determine if the fix is improving the results and/or lowering barriers to implementation. The most felicitous option is that the improvement cycle results exceed the threshold to implement that step. In this fortunate condition, the designer may be ready to move to the next step or even to implement the entire SIP.

At the end, decisions must be taken and actions must be initiated: implement, revise, or drop. At some point, the process has been improved enough that implementation of a step can go ahead, even though it may not produce a perfect result. The challenge is to determine if you have reached the limits of the D3A3 improvement model, with it now reaching a performance plateau and signaling the designer that it is time to move on to full implementation of a good-enough solution. If the designer is satisfied that the impact/effort/yield formulation has topped out, reached the needed threshold, and is ready, the step should be implemented. If there is continued disconcerting uncertainty and more ideas about improving the intervention, the designer should feel safe recommending another improvement model test run. And if the maximum of assurance about impact/yield/risk has been reached and yet the designer is unable either to go forward or to envision further improvements, the planner has the answer they need: it is best to drop that step and even to reconsider the feasibility of the SIP.

As improvement cycles proceed, the planner should be going back and forth from each step to consider the SIP as an integrated whole. The steps are interactive and continuous, building toward an output that drives achievement of the goals. If any step falls short of meeting the criteria for implementation, the designer should consider the feasibility of the SIP itself. In a tight causal chain of steps, failure of one step endangers the entire SIP.

Second Small Group Meeting (Two Hours)

Use this group meeting to review the steps, expected problems, and proposed solutions in the implementation of the group's SIP. Each student presents their step in the implementation of the plan, summarizes the three Ds and As improvement process, including proposed outcomes and measures of performance, explains what they propose to mitigate the major problems, states the expected outputs, and describes their level of confidence in achieving the result. The group discusses and critiques each step in the causal chain, and then works together to confirm the SIP.

The goal is for the group to finalize their SIP and prepare the plan and their overall goal for change for presentation to their colleagues. The objective is to present the goals of their system change in their country and describe why the SIP will achieve it. The group will create a storyboard (Box 6.4) to present their SIP at the large group meeting.

Box 6.4: STORY BOARD FORMAT

System improvement plan title
Team members
Statement of problem
Description of the proposed solution
    The goal and why it is an important improvement.
    Description of the change process—what, where, when, how.
    Will it work? What are the major uncertainties and downside risks?
Plan of work
    Describe how the work will be done.

What will be the intervention?
What are the key measures of success?
How will the results data be collected?
How will the data be analyzed?
Proposed impact, effort, and risk
How is it an improvement? Answer to "So what? Who cares? What difference will it make?"
Effort (feasibility, time, money) and risks of failure.
Why this is deserving of your support?

LARGE GROUP PRESENTATION OF IMPLEMENTATION PLANS

In the final step of this section, each SIP will be presented in a meeting of all course participants. Students in their small group of should present as a unit. Each country group will generally follow the story board format, describing their country's setting, presenting the problem and goals, and explaining their SIP. Each will have 10 minutes to present, followed by 5 minutes of reaction, questions, critique, and suggestions. If the schedule can be adhered to, three subgroups can present per hour, and up to nine groups can present and vote in a morning or afternoon session.

CHAPTER 7

Insights From Systems Thinking

The significant problems we have cannot be solved at the same level of thinking with which we created them.

—Albert Einstein

Systems thinking is a distinctive and nuanced way to conceptualize a health system. This view discloses levels of complexity, interactions, and interdependency that a static view does not easily offer. Systems thinking can provide new insights into how a system works and generate ideas about how to solve its problems. Understanding health systems in their systems theory complexity reveals incipient trade-offs, log jams, and unintended consequences that together are a formidable force of resistance to change.

Three high-level insights can be taken from this workbook's look at a health system from a systems thinking perspective.

1. Every health system suffers from one of systems theory's classic descriptive models called *"The Tragedy of the Commons,"* in which a scarce resource is consumed when a collective benefit (e.g., health insurance) is subsidized and its price to the user is less than the cost to produce it. This insight emerges from the perspective of systems dynamics.
2. When viewed from the perspective of value-for-money, health systems face *competing objectives about the benefits and performance* it should produce. The objectives are satisfying individual's expectations and

demands for their own medical care, providing healthcare as a funda-mental right of all citizens regardless of ability to pay, and improving the health of the nation. Balancing between these three, and with the added objective of national affordability of the costs of healthcare, is the core problem that must be solved if sustainable high-value healthcare is to endure at a national level.

3. Underpinning the three distinctive objectives are differences in values and mental maps reflecting how citizens see the world, rationalize its processes, and interpret events. Balancing between and among these objectives calls for very different thinking and learning approaches to the design and implementation of change. This type of system change requires revealing and then reframing these mental maps. We discuss *Model 2 thinking that enables double-loop learning*, which is required when confronting *second-order change*. The latter describes problems where it is necessary to redesign human perceptions in order for change to lead to improvement.

APPLYING SYSTEMS THINKING AND DISCOVERING THE TRAGEDY OF THE COMMONS

In exploring The Tragedy of the Commons, we discuss how insights can be used from systems dynamics—an approach that has been used to con-ceptualize and model complex systems and apply systems thinking in practice.[1]

Systems Dynamics

In handling high detail and complexity, systems dynamics is a powerful tool with many applications. It helps in understanding social structures, in much the same way as engineering principles help understanding me-chanical systems. In systems dynamics, an organization or system and its respective environment (context) is viewed as a complex whole of interrelated and interdependent parts, rather than separate entities (Box 7.1). A systems view of a health system and the application of systems dy-namics enables us to visualize and understand the major design challenges it faces.

Box 7.1: SYSTEMS DYNAMICS

System Dynamics portrays a real or proposed system and its inputs and outputs in a special kind of interactive flow diagram that simplifies and maps the dynamics of a complex system using interacting feedback loops. Structures and flows are characterized by a set of patterns, which describe and identify many of the common behaviors in a system, including internal balancing feedback loops and time delays

The interrelationships presented in this format show distinctive patterns with important consequences that affect results. These patterns fall into typical classic models, which are called *archetypes*. Knowing the type of archetypes has led to a better understanding of the nonlinear behavior of dynamic complex systems over time. In *The Fifth Discipline Field Book*, these archetypes are presented as accessible tools which managers use to quickly construct credible and consistent hypotheses about the governing forces in their system.[2] Discerning the archetypes that describe a system helps one to clarify the mental models underlying the system.

System dynamics modeling and the use of archetypes can help in understanding the state of play of a system. The framework we use to conceptualize a health system in this workbook has systems thinking at its core and considers dynamic complexity and the interaction of the health system within its context. Systems dynamics modeling enables hypothesis testing and generation of scenarios, as well as enhanced joint thinking, group learning, and shared understanding of problems. This joint thinking process can be combined with qualitative or quantitative systems dynamics modeling to simulate system behavior under explicit assumptions. Systems dynamics modeling can be used to demonstrate relationships, potential interactions, and possible outcomes under different scenarios or to quantify the magnitude of potential effects with different policy scenarios.[3]

Systems dynamics modeling has also been used in the health system setting for hypothesis testing, in generation of what-if analyses of different policy scenarios, to develop shared understanding of problems, to enhance joint thinking, and to facilitate group learning.[4–7]

Health Insurance From a Systems Dynamics Perspective

For most of its long history, medical care was a relatively simple system: a market transaction between doctor and patient. A sick patient sought help from a doctor when ill. They explicitly or implicitly agreed on the benefits and determined the cost. When the doctor provided the service, he received the payment from the patient.

There are many reasons why this was never an ideal market transaction, but the model endured in its simple form because the medical benefits were deemed to be of value, and for a typical consultation the cost to the user was generally low. However, in this model, healthcare access was determined by the ability to pay rather than by need. Many who could not afford to pay for a doctor could not access healthcare when ill and suffered as a result. This was a fundamental flaw in the model that needed to be fixed.

As we outlined in Chapter 3, several momentous design changes occurred in almost all health systems, mostly in the 20th century. First and foremost, as medical care became more effective, complicated, and expensive, populations in work groups or nationals banded together and pooled their money to protect themselves against the financial risk of illness and thus to ensure broad access. The idea was that the need for care was an uncommon event and that those who were fortunate enough to remain well would contribute to a pool that could be used to pay for those who required care. Insurance was born as a concept.

It was not long before insurance was widely extended. Most countries came steadily to the conclusion that healthcare was a basic human right (articulated in the United Nations Declaration of Human Rights adopted by the UN General Assembly in 1948)[8] and 'health for all' became a goal set by the World Health Organization for all countries[9]. It followed that all citizens deserved the right to be covered by insurance and protected from their healthcare costs, which would be paid out of the common insurance pool contributed to by individuals, businesses, or through taxation. The responsibility for meeting the cost of healthcare services shifted from the patient to the insurance pool. With this arrangement the cost to the individual was as low as 'free at the point of use' as in England, or at least subsidized to varying degrees in different countries and ranges of medical services. Businesses, unions, and then nations either provided healthcare insurance, or they actually built, provided, and ran a ready-made health system.

What was covered by the pool expanded over time. At first, insurance was limited to a narrow set of benefits consisting primarily of hospital care. Insurance coverage was limited to serious, urgent, expensive, or life-threatening illnesses. But the success of the concept of insurance stimulated its gradual extension to lower cost services, such as visits for minor illness, prevention and screening, and simple tests and procedures. Insurance gradually expanded to cover almost all health services used by the pooled population. Most nations endorsed the idea that everyone should have accessible and affordable care and directed resources to create their own health system to deliver primary as well as advanced care to all.

Today, almost all high-income countries operate from this generic model of benefits, costs, and payments guaranteed by health insurance (or tax financing), a far cry from when an individual paid directly for the services they received. This design guarantees every citizen access to individual medical services when they believe they need it, pools the resources to pay for the costs this service generates, and subsidizes the price to the individual at the point of use. Most modern health systems in middle- and high-income countries are built around this design of universal health coverage funded predominantly by health insurance or general taxation. The design reflects common societal priorities and choices among consumers and political leaders. Comparatively, although it still is a national service, public health support has withered and trails far behind what we spend on individual medical care.

Upward pressure on healthcare costs: a symptom of The Tragedy of the Commons

The emergence of the health insurance model has added a third party to that original market transaction between doctor and patient—an insurance pool that is a collective resource covering a whole population. The health system shifted from a simple patient-doctor transaction to one in which there are now three actors—the patient, the provider, and the payer (that funds and usually manages the pooled resources). The patient is protected from the full cost of care. The payer can be a government, an agency (such as a social insurance fund), a private insurance company, or an individual working through an insurance function that can be governmental, private, or some combination. The payers are responsible for covering the costs of care, managing the risk of over-utilization and protecting the common pool of financial resources available to pay for the provider services delivered to patients.

Let us examine that design challenge that leads to tensions in balancing the goals of improving health and satisfaction while managing costs. The challenge starts with a laudable goal: a nation wants to provide healthcare as a right and to share the financial expense of that care for an individual in a common pool across the entire population. That is, the resource is pooled with the understanding that it will be used for those who become sick; the cost to an individual who needs and gets care is underwritten by those in the pool who pay-in but don't need the care because they remain healthy.

This distinctive pattern in healthcare is a classic Systems Dynamic archetype—"The Tragedy of the Commons." In 1968 ecologist Garrett

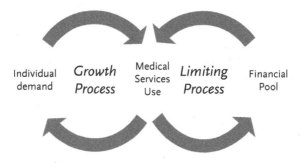

Figure 7.1 The Tragedy of the Commons archetype.

Hardin described the general phenomenon in which rational self-interest acts in such a way as to drive overuse and deplete a common, shared resource. He called this "The Tragedy of the Commons,"[10] using the name coined by William Forster Lloyd who first discovered the economic principles in the mid-19th century.[11] They both describe this as a circumstance in which a collectively supported village Commons was open to all for grazing. A herdsman had an incentive to overuse the resource because the benefit to him and his herd exceeded his cost, since the cost was shared by all. Soon all herdsmen over-grazed the grass, and the resource itself was destroyed. This structural flaw is well-known to systems experts as a trap; they still call the archetype The Tragedy of the Commons.

The healthcare application of The Tragedy of the Commons systems archetype consists of a reinforcing loop and a corresponding balancing, or limiting, loop (Figure 7.1). Left on its own, the reinforcing loop will eventually be slowed by the limiting process. In healthcare, the insurance pool would run out and the benefits would stop.

Almost all health systems in high-income countries, with their current design assumptions, are examples of The Tragedy of the Commons. In middle-income and high-income countries, the trajectory of healthcare costs has been persistently upward for many decades, well exceeding the rates of economic growth as measured by Gross Domestic Product. Why might that be? Of course, much is the result of advances in the process of care. But also, because the individual is sheltered from the cost (which can create a *moral hazard*, since an individual who does not bear the full risk of paying for care has no financial disincentive to moderate their use of unnecessary healthcare services), system overuse is likely (Figure 7.2). A full coverage, collective insurance system structurally encourages consumers to over-use the common resource of universal health insurance. When a portion of the use is inappropriate or unnecessary, there is relatively

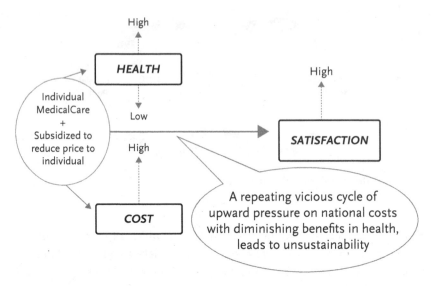

Figure 7.2 Individual medical care and costs.

little change in health. This dynamic creates waste and draws down the insurance pool.

The Tragedy of the Commons is built into the generic health system design. It is a characteristic that, coupled with the growth of technology, virtually guarantees that any population with subsidized universal care that aims to provide all healthcare services and interventions without priority setting will find their system ultimately to be unsustainable.

Healthcare is different than most other insurance businesses, such as car insurance, that collect money in advance and pool risk. Medical care is subject, more than others, to moral hazard. Healthcare, like all insurance, has a built-in tension between the individual choice to use and safeguarding the collective benefit. However, in car insurance, for example, much of the risk is predictable and can be priced easily into premiums. Financial incentives can be used to reward nonusers but would generally be inappropriate in discouraging healthcare use. Moreover, no one wants to have a car accident, so claiming car insurance is both a clear endpoint and also not an outcome that people want.

Receiving and paying for care is no longer a straight-forward consumer decision (for better or for worse). No longer does a simple buyer–seller transaction set the market and consumer rules to balance supply and demand, adjust prices, and stimulate innovation. Rather, the new structure puts the doctor on the same side as the patient, aligning the interests of both in providing care that is paid from the collective public insurance pool.

We illustrate this new buyer–seller transaction in Figure 7.3. Not all that care is of high value.

In addition to the incentives built into The Tragedy of the Commons, the alignment of the patient and provider further accelerates demand. Patients expect to get the care they want (which may not always be the same as the care they need). Doctors, with their natural motivation to heal, want to do the most they can for each patient, make the patient happy, increase their own income, and adhere to their professional oath to advocate for what the patient wants. Doctors and patients are partners in raising demand. When patients experience no major cost constraint and are encouraged by their medical professional and when the provider of care making the recommendation has financial and other incentives to overorder diagnostic tests or provide nonvalue-adding healthcare interventions, the combination acts like an accelerant to the underlying tendency of the system to overuse the available pool of resources.

The power dynamics in this model favor the consumer and provider of care. Instead of the patient experiencing the price for the service, they are now sheltered from the direct costs. The providers are compensated for their services from a prepaid or prospectively budgeted collective pool, yet the payer generally holds the risks and costs for overutilization. The dynamic has naturally shifted leverage toward the provider and patient, who both benefit from the delivery of care, while the payer lacks information,

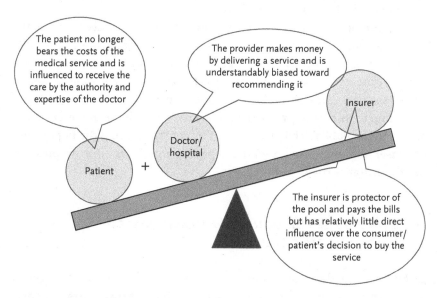

Figure 7.3 The service transaction favors buyer over payer.

often is involved after the fact, and is distrusted by both provider and patient. In this arrangement, the payers have become identified as the withholders or blockers of care—or as agents of rationing.

Addressing The Tragedy of the Commons

What to do about the basic flaw—The Tragedy of the Commons? How do nations take on the vicious cycle of The Tragedy of the Commons and continue to provide healthcare for all regardless of ability to pay? How do they block the archetype's ill effects and slow, eventually stop, or even reverse it? Left unchecked, The Tragedy of the Commons will eventually correct itself, although late in the process when much damage has already been done.

With emerging limitations of the resources in the pool, many nations have already begun to act to preserve the societal right to universal availability to high-quality healthcare services. Most health systems in middle- and high-income countries have already encountered and attempted to constrain, mitigate, or delay the effect of The Tragedy of the Commons. The system planners' greatest challenge is to fix the major design limitations and threats from The Tragedy of the Commons. Some have failed, most notably because of poorly designed regulation that leads to market failure, passive payers that act as administrative pass-through entities rather than strategic purchasers, absence of meaningful priority-setting, and inadequate individual citizen responsibility.

Intervening early with design changes can mitigate or even reverse the potentially malign effects of The Tragedy of the Commons. A set of available policy interventions include regulation, use of market forces, or persuasion (directed towards healthcare service providers or citizens to modify their behavior). For example, the designer could set limits on service use, price it up to its cost of production or beyond through the use of tariffs, or appeal to the public's civic mindedness by communicating the importance of conserving the pooled resource as part of a national effort to preserve health insurance coverage for all.

ACHIEVING VALUE-FOR-MONEY IN A HEALTH SYSTEM BY BROADENING ITS GOALS

Clearly getting the most value-for-money is an aspiration all national health systems share. Few countries would claim that their current models are delivering the level of value that citizens deserve from the hard-won money they spend directly or indirectly on healthcare. From the perspective of getting more health for its investment, a country surely would want to optimize its system to produce the most health from the financial resources it has chosen to spend.

There are many definitions of value-for-money and its components. One of the early definitions by the National Audit Office in the United Kingdom developed in the 1990s for the National Health System, has considered value-for-money in terms of economy (minimizing the cost of resources used), efficiency (relationship between outputs and the resources used to produce them), effectiveness (extent to which intended objectives of a service are achieved), and cost-effectiveness (extent to which resources are used to achieve outcomes).[12] More recently, value in healthcare has been defined by Michael Porter and Elizabeth Tiesberg as health outcomes achieved that matter to patients relative to the cost of achieving those outcomes.[13] In their view, the determination of value-for-money is the framework for making decisions about what care is worth paying for. They argue, using the US context as the basis of their analysis, that competition between providers of care for the custom of patients should be enhanced; better application of market forces, they argue, would lead to better outcomes, more health, and lower prices.

These definitions of the benefits of a health system are instrumental but incomplete. The definitions focus on medical interventions and primarily consider clinical results as the measure of benefit. But these are not all the benefits that people hope for. These definitions have not adequately considered citizen satisfaction from the perspective of either their personal care or equity of access to that care.

A national health system's achievement of overall value-for-money is usually based on the health benefits they achieve for the money they spend. Value, as measured in the term *value-for-money*, is usually limited to health outcomes, services, or benefits. In this section, we make the case that the current concept of health value is too restrictive and needs to be widened to include each country's unique definition of satisfaction.

Clinical results are not the only concern for people when they think about the value they receive from their health system. Citizens have expectations of their health system and want these expectations to be met to their satisfaction. The definition of satisfaction should include the elements that reflect what that nation's citizenry assumes their health system should deliver. In setting goals to enhance value, a nation must define *health* and *satisfaction* in its own terms to begin determining how to achieve it.

Measuring the success of a health system depends on adding *satisfaction* to the country's ability to enhance the two goals of improving the health

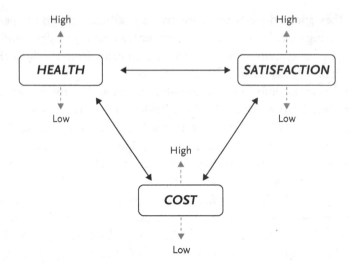

Figure 7.4 Balancing national goals.

of the nation at a cost the nation can afford (Figure 7.4). The design of the system has a profound influence on optimizing the balance between these three national goals.

A New Value Proposition That Expands Its Definition to Include Satisfaction

If it is to serve as a useful parameter of health system performance, satisfaction needs further explicit definition and specification. Satisfaction is a feeling of fulfilment that is enhanced by meeting or exceeding citizen expectations. But in a health system, people want different things. Expectations vary among different population segments.

We propose that there are two basic clusters of expectations that influence satisfaction in individuals and nations. In Figure 7.5 we present a schematic model in which the measure of satisfaction displays this duality in the way citizens gauge it. In one grouping of expectations, the personal experience of care is paramount. For the other, concerns about equity and social solidarity are foremost. Underneath each set of expectations lie differing values, mental maps, and governing beliefs. The two orientations of course coexist in most countries. But we believe that one or the other tends to predominate.

Some nations believe that individualism and self-interest is the way society works best. The mental map that influences the expectations of a

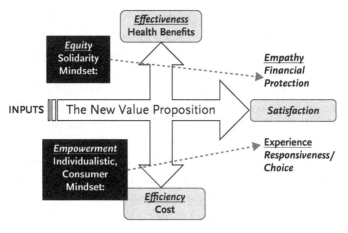

Figure 7.5 The six E's: a new value proposition for a health system.
Adapted from Moore G, Quelch J, and Boudreau E. *Choice Matters*. New York, NY: Oxford University Press. 2018.

consumer-centered experience highly rates individualism and the freedom to choose. These countries generally share the mindset that people have to deserve what they get. This feeling is especially strong in countries like the United States that are consumer-oriented and market-driven.

The individually oriented group reflects that citizens want their personal experience to be the dominant goal. They expect their healthcare to be responsive to their perceived needs, available to them upon demand, a good experience as a consumer, and structured so they can exercise choice over what they receive. They expect to have a really good experience with their own care.

The other group emphasizes a cluster of expectations that are communitarian. They value equity and fairness. They see social solidarity and concern for others as measures that define success. The societal values that support care-for-all regardless of ability to pay reflect an underlying shared belief about what is just. They care about and are empathic to the plight of others. In this perspective, all citizens share a view of the need for collective fairness, the value of working together in the interests of the community, and the importance of solidarity and shared values. Citizenship means caring for and about the entire population, not just themselves.

A group with these communitarian values will have a strong belief in equity of access to healthcare, empathy toward those in need, and fairness for all regardless of ability to pay. This grouping emphasizes adequate financial protection to enable all citizens to access their health system. The expectations are that access to care is a public good. They take pride in being on the team in such a system. These citizens are likely to rate their satisfaction with their national system as poor if they perceive the system as failing to provide care to others that is as good as that which they receive themselves.

Of course, citizens in all developed countries want their health system to satisfy both clusters of expectations. As patients, they are individual consumers of medical services. They quite naturally want those services to be accessible and affordable, deliver good results for the personal problem for which they sought care, and give them a satisfying experience as a consumer of care. But a second communitarian force tugs at citizens and colors their satisfaction as well: healthcare should be accessible to all. Meeting both these expectations is espoused by most people as important.

Nations differ in how well they strike a balance between the two sets of expectations. Countries vary in their achievement of citizens' underlying priorities regarding what constitutes satisfaction with their health system. Figure 7.6 illustrates how three countries differ in the integration of the two sets of expectations. England has achieved a good balance, while the United States falls short on equity and fairness. Denmark underperforms on individual choice. The model also shows that countries can enhance overall satisfaction by improving performance in both sets of measured satisfaction, moving to the right and up in the chart.

We believe that one or the other perspective tends to predominate at both the individual and national level at this time. National populations hold a mix of these two sets of expectations, but each country has its own attraction to and leans toward one or the other view of satisfaction. Countries with strong solidarity and sense of equity are biased to be supportive of a

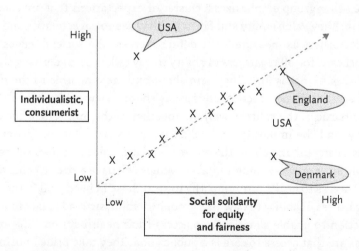

Figure 7.6 Illustrating national balancing of individual consumerist and social solidarity.

system that provides insurance and care that covers everyone. Countries with a strong individual consumer orientation are inherently less likely to criticize their system for not covering everyone and more likely to be upset when their personal services are not able to meet their expectations of a satisfying consumer experience.

Nevertheless, the aspiration of all health systems should be to achieve high value by maximizing the health of the nation, attaining satisfaction with *both* the individual and collective health perspectives, and doing both at the lowest and most sustainable national cost.

These two views of satisfaction compete for resources. Individual care and universal insurance coverage costs are escalating. Consumers expect to get more and are dissatisfied when services are not available or subsidized. Extending care to all consumes resources that might otherwise be spent on maximizing benefits and satisfaction with individual care. Where the care is free and based on need, the drain on the common financial resource to pay for it is high. When resources are constrained, designing a system that satisfies both sets of expectations and health needs and yet stays within affordable costs is of critical importance.

In Figure 7.7, we present a framework to illustrate that countries can achieve a balance between individual and collective satisfaction and that

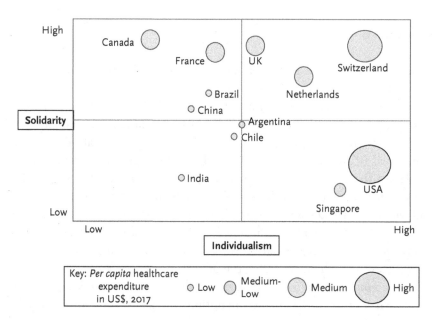

Figure 7.7 The balance of individual and communitarian interests in a health system by healthcare expenditure.

some accomplish this at lower cost. Value-for-money increases through better design and management.

England is an example of a country that does relatively well in meeting both sets of satisfaction-related expectations and does so for comparatively low cost. Their healthcare model provides universal care for all (through the National Health Service [NHS]) in a very efficient, capacity-constrained, but well-regarded delivery system. Its expenditure on healthcare is relatively low. Yet the NHS remains revered as a national treasure and is rated one of the most popular health systems.[14] The design of the NHS appears to create value-for-money and is a source of national pride. In 2017, the United Kingdom spent £2,989 per person on healthcare and 9.6% of gross domestic product, at about the median expenditure for other country members of the Organisation for Economic Co-operation and Development, which was £2,913 per person.[15]

Switzerland and the Netherlands, which also achieve high satisfaction in balancing the sets of goals, spent much more per capita (£5,417 and £3,907, respectively) and as a proportion of gross domestic product (11.9% and 10.1%, respectively) than England on healthcare in 2017.[20] Better design of their system would be required were they to decide to constrain overall health system spending while maintaining or even improving national measures of health and satisfaction.

The Balancing Act

The design of the health system has a profound influence on maximizing overall value-for-money. A national health system's performance is determined by the achievement of a sustainable balance among the three national goals: health of the nation, the cost to the nation, and the ultimate level of satisfaction of its citizens, given the differing expectations we have described (Figure 7.8). Every nation will strive to produce the most possible health and satisfaction at whatever price it can afford to pay for its health system. Population level goals such as overall health and care-for-all will interact and compete with those of understandably self-interested individuals focusing on their own needs. The third variable to be solved for in the value-for-money equation is the absolute cost and sustainability of the system as a whole, including the opportunity cost—what other things citizens must give up for what is spent on healthcare. The design of the system has a profound influence on optimizing the three national goals.

The route to improving value in the health system is to define more precisely what *it* means to a nation and to determine the best balance for them

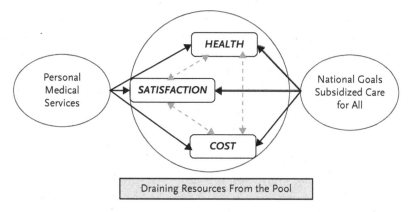

Figure 7.8 Individual care and national goals—a balancing act.

between the benefits—overall health, personal care services, and social co-hesiveness with access to care for all (medical care as a human right), and financial sustainability—given the ceiling of resources available as deter-mined by national productivity and allocation to healthcare among other national priorities.

UNDERSTANDING THE COMPLEXITY OF CHANGE

Change comes in three flavors. The first two are called *first-order and second-order change*. The third is reconceptualization.

First-order change is a fix for a problem that is within an existing system; it is intended to bring the system under better control. First-order change is the solution to a problem that requires us to do more—or less—of some-thing we are already doing. It does not require changing the underlying structure of the system itself nor the values and frames of those involved. It is relatively easily implemented. An example is the change in tempera-ture that is triggered by system feedback when a thermostat detects that it is cold and sends a turn-on signal to a heater.

We learn the basic tools of first-order change thinking early in the first few years of life, as a means to guide us to effective responses to our immediate threats and needs. It is called Model 1 thinking, and it is our default mode of thinking. We develop mental maps, which are subcon-scious representations of how the world works. These mental maps make it possible to understand and interpret our experiences automatically, act quickly, and efficiently navigate our surroundings. It is how we are biologi-cally primed to think and act.

Model 1 thinking is handy and quick. It is built around mental shortcuts that are right at hand when we need them to make a quick judgment and act fast. But Model 1 thinking is prone to bias and error when it is used for more complex problems, as described by Daniel Kahneman in his book *Thinking Fast and Slow*.[16] Model 1 thinking and its educational partner, single-loop learning,[17] are the way that most individuals think, communicate, and act—even though they may espouse differently. It is our default mode of reflection and action in most situations, including second-order change, where it is usually ineffective.

Model 1 thinking convinces the user that they are right, seals up their behavior from scrutiny from themselves or others, and makes it nondiscussable. It is based on our looking good, being right, and making implicit assumptions about the motivation of others, all the while not recognizing that we are actually thinking this way when asked how we make decisions. Model 1 thinking lacks the capacity to be reflective—it is incapable of deep questioning, thinking, and learning. Without such learning capability, a system is stuck in Model 1 thinking, where goals, values, frameworks, and, to a significant extent, strategies are taken for granted and cannot be influenced in the change process.

By contrast, second-order problems require changing the system. Solutions to second-order change problems modify the existing system structure and force people to rethink how they interpret and frame their new experience. Governing variables and mental maps must themselves be the subject of inquiry and analysis. Health system change is almost always second order.

Resolving these complex second-order problems requires what is called Model 2 thinking, and it is associated with double-loop learning. Single-loop learning is ineffective. In this perspective on complex systems, human behavior is considered to be a major barrier to learning, implementing change, and making improvement. Solving this kind of problem requires a different way of thinking that enables new ways of learning to understand, examine, and change values, beliefs, attitudes, and communication style.

A Systems Model for Change

Whether your system improvement plan (SIP) change requires single- or double-loop learning strongly influences how hard it will be to implement and succeed. Clearly achieving a new state of balance between alternative understandings of health system goals is a second-order change problem. Knowing the class of the problem you are dealing with is important because the choice of modes of implementation differ in fundamental ways. The underlying typology of your SIP influences its design, clarifies its vulnerabilities as a plan, and determines the approach needed for implementation.

We believe that there are three major classes of systems dynamics problems—first order, second order, and paradigmatic change (think of this as *disorder*). Which one describes your SIP determines the scope of effort and learning you need to achieve a successful outcome. The three systems problems classes are illustrated in a schematic adapted from Argyris and Schön[23] (Figure 7.9). The three classes of problem types are not mutually exclusive; there are often overlapping elements. Each represents a different category of problem.

First-order change problems (those that exist within the existing structure and do not need people to change behaviors) need only Model 1 thinking and single-loop learning to solve what are primarily mechanistic problems. This simplest change classification (labeled as *react*) of implementation is instrumental. That is, the change is not influenced by the values, beliefs, mental maps, or attitudes of the participants. The system failures are in design or execution.

The learning needed to solve first-order change problems is single-loop. It is mechanistic. The challenge is largely one of mechanical design or logistical management. Model 2 thinking is unnecessary. In fixing a problem like this, the planner relies on engineering types of interventions, where the fixes are operational. Mitigation is often quick and economical. Except

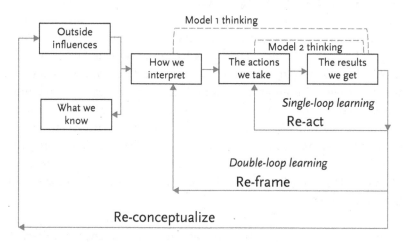

Figure 7.9 Classifying the type of systems fix.

when solving simple instrumental problems, Model 1 thinking is of limited usefulness in health system change.

A health system's most important challenges represent second-order change. Second-order change problems modify the existing system structure. Health system problems call for solutions that influence people's personal and interpersonal behavior. People are forced to question their personal mental maps regarding health system goals and how they interpret and frame their new experience. Significant health system change almost always encounters competing interests, conflicting preferences, self-serving defensive behavior, and differing convictions about what action to take. This type of problem requires Model 2 thinking and double-loop learning.

Model 2 thinking and double-loop learning are critical skills in complex health systems facing second-order change. Advanced learning is required to solve second-order change problems. Reflection-in-action is needed to resolve underlying tensions that arise from competing interests, mental maps, and theories of action.

Reframing is a necessary skill to solve problems that involve these human interactions and values. Successful improvement in this class of problem requires what Argyris and Schön call double-loop learning.[23] This type of learning entails understanding people's mental map of their lived world and examining and reframing their, and one's own, attitudes, deep knowledge of themselves, and what Argyris and Schön call theory-in-action.[23] A theory-in-action is the real rationale for how individuals actually act in response to change, and it reflects the mental model they use to frame how they interpret and respond to the specific problem they are confronting.

Double-loop learning requires reframing a person's mindset—individual beliefs, mental maps, and theories-in-action. The learning involves understanding others' and one's own interests, biases, theories of how things work, and mental models that lead us to decide what is fair or not. This is hard to do. But change is rarely successful in this class of systems dynamics problem without applying an individual and organizational model of open, active inquiry about underlying motivations and examination of how people think about their work and behavior. The systems expert Peter Senge designates an organization capable of this skilled inquiry to be a learning organization.[18] To implement an SIP that requires a change in stakeholder behavior, Senge would argue that the task calls for a learning systems approach.[25]

The third category, conceptual challenges, are those in which the problems are disorderly. This type of systems challenge manifests as results that can't be ascribed to either mechanistic design problems or to human conflicts arising from differences in mind-set and assumptions. The breakdown pushes beyond what we know. Our current understandings, mental maps, and know-how cannot explain the problem and its possible solutions. Conceptual change problems often reveal themselves through baffling or complete surprises, well outside our ability to understand. The system may face an existential threat or major context shift (such as a pandemic, new technologies or a dramatic societal alteration in values) that creates the need and opportunity for entirely new thinking.

Reconceptualization is a paradigm shift. Conceptual change requires a new way of understanding healthcare and its problems, generating unfamiliar new mental models and theories-in-action. The change cannot be formulated from within the existing know-how, mental constructs, and knowledge. Conceptual problems are disruptive and stimulate solutions that shift existing mental maps and theories-in-action.

When a system fails to produce what its population and environment need, it will eventually stop functioning. The result creates vague dissatisfaction among the participants and a sense that there is a mismatch between what the system is producing in outputs and outcomes and what the context calls for. Here there is often a deep gulf between the mental map, knowledge, and knowhow of those inside the system and the consumer of its outputs, an archetypal systems flaw or vicious cycle that makes the system unstable or unsustainable, or a technologic breakthrough that creates the opportunity to deliver what citizens want. The remedy for this class of system problem is deeper and more fundamental— it requires reconceptualization of purpose, product, and process as well as modifications of belief, values, and mental maps to align with the new paradigm.

SECOND-ORDER CHANGE AS THE HEALTH SYSTEM NORM

As discussed, the new value-for-money model contains two distinctive frameworks of expectations lurking in the national psyche. Adapting to trade-offs and accepting the reality of compromise requires double-loop learning and reframing. When change addresses beliefs and mindsets as different as individualistic consumer-orientation and social solidarity and equity, both must be understood and held simultaneously in the new values framework needed to enjoy a sustainable, fair, and effective health system.

In our own experience, most worthwhile change is second order, requiring a significant change in the way things are done in a system. The vast majority of students following the educational design curriculum in this workbook have chosen goals or outcomes that are Model 2 changes. To design and implement a Model 2 change requires double-loop learning in its implementation. The measure of its success is sufficient public cohesiveness to support the actionable change.

Double-loop learning is a high-effort, high-skill undertaking. Resolving conflicts of interests and values is no easy task. In the next chapter, we will discuss the importance of high levels of cohesiveness in an organization or a system to work out differences when implementing an SIP with social elements. Double-loop learning requires active, often uncomfortable inquiry.

SUMMARY

Systems thinking has shed some light on understanding how a given health system works and what it will take to implement change that could make it better. First, The Tragedy of the Commons was identified as the most important single design challenge to planners. To increase value-for-money, any change starts by finding a way to increase the cost-effectiveness of the benefits that are covered and slow down expenditures on the system. Second, each country's definition of value-for-money is unique but all are attempting to deliver a mix of the three benefits—overall health of its public, individual care and service, and collective value of a public system of insurance to give every citizen access to needed care regardless of ability to pay. Third, the complex changes we need are likely to require double-loop learning, in which conflicts and differing values and beliefs need to be surfaced and managed.

These are formidable challenges. No one country has yet effectively solved how to perfectly balance the goals of health, individual and collective satisfaction, and affordability. What we do know is that the solution will call on skills, knowledge, and attitude changes that have been hard to achieve.

CHAPTER 8

Implementing a Change—Adoption and Diffusion

It ought to be remembered that there is nothing more difficult to take in hand, more perilous to conduct, or more uncertain in its success, than to take the lead in the introduction of a new order of things. Because the innovator has for enemies all those who have done well under the old conditions and lukewarm defenders in those who may do well under the new. This coolness arises partly from fear of the opponents, who have the laws on their side, and partly from the incredulity of men, who do not readily believe in new things until they have had a long experience of them

—Niccolò Machiavelli

Innovations and new policies must be implemented and reach sufficient scale to have an impact on health outcomes. Even when financing is available, the uptake of innovations and new policies remains low, especially in the countries and populations that need them most. Indeed, it has proven particularly challenging to implement innovations in health systems, even when there is compelling evidence for their cost-effectiveness.[1]

The achievement of sustainable improvement in a health system requires, of course, a good plan that is executed well. We refer to the adoption of a new policy or an innovative plan (and hereafter for simplicity we will use the terms system improvement plan [SIP], a policy, or an innovation interchangeably, as they all are intended to produce change) as the goal to establish a foothold of users who undertake, as Everett Rogers said in his seminal work on diffusion of innovation, "to make full use of an innovation as the best course of action available."[2p5] Diffusion is the dispersion of innovation. It occurs when "an innovation is communicated through certain channels over time among members of a social system."[2p5] The objective of diffusion is to scale-up an SIP until it is sustainable at an acceptable cost.

Achieving change and improvement depend on both adoption and scaling up to achieve impact from an improvement. Adoption of an SIP requires sufficient uptake by a risk-taking, first-mover group to establish the credibility of the change. This group will prove that the change works (or not), is an improvement, and is acceptable. Diffusion is the spread of the innovation beyond a first-adopter, risk-taking group to others who are more risk-averse and question change. The latter take a wait-and-see approach.

One of the reasons that second-order change efforts at redesign falter is a simplistic view of the course of change. Adoption and diffusion of innovations are frequently considered to be linear processes, which might work with first-order change problems but is unlikely to succeed with second-order change. Prevailing approaches shaped by this linear view in many health systems have typically focused on *push models*, where changes are initiated without much attention paid to the complex system into which they are introduced. In these models, the underlying assumption is that by merely increasing resource inputs, the desired improvements in outputs and outcomes will happen. All too often this is the prevailing approach in health systems. However, as earlier discussed, the introduction of innovations or new policies into a complex adaptive system upsets the equilibrium and causes such systems to oppose the interventions, leading to resistance. Consequently, many well-conceived ideas fail to be adopted and never achieve the intended results.

INFLUENCES ON IMPLEMENTATION

The literature shows that adoption and diffusion of innovations in health systems are influenced by multiple factors that interact as part of the structure of a dynamic system.[3] These factors include, as examples

- How the innovation is perceived by adopters,[4] such as clinicians.[5]
- The nature and perception of the problem being addressed.
- Prevailing cultural norms, beliefs, and values of the key actors and institutions within the adoption system[6] in particular professional groups and opinion leaders.[7,8]
- The complexity of the innovation.[9–12]
- Institutional practices in organizations.[13]
- The institutional logic of key stakeholders involved in the innovation adoption.[14]

- Health system factors, such as organizational design, regulatory environment, financing, provider payment systems, and service delivery models in use.[15,16]
- Broader contextual factors, such as sociocultural norms, societal beliefs, and political values.[17–19]

In addition, adoption and diffusion of innovations or new policies in health systems are shaped by factors related to the learning capacity of the adoption system. These include

- Social networks,[20] systems, and structures that enable learning within an organization.[21]
- The absorptive capacity for new knowledge within the adopting organization or individuals.[22,23]

As discussed, every health system, where these factors and elements are interconnected and interdependent, exhibits characteristics of complex systems.[24,25] Thus, when introducing an innovation in a health system, it is necessary to take a systems view to ensure its timely adoption and diffusion.

THE STUDENT WORK PLAN

The behavioral learning objective for this chapter is for each student to formulate a plan for implementing their SIP. In this exercise, all students in the course will be working on their own SIP developed at the end of Chapter 6 of this volume. There will be one small group discussion and a final large group meeting for presentation and feedback.

In their independent study activity, each student will go through the stepwise process of developing the implementation plan following the model we describe and prepare to present their plan in the small group meeting. In that meeting, the small group will consolidate their thinking and prepare a short presentation of their plan to present at the final all-group meeting.

USING THE 7CS MODEL

Successfully maneuvering an SIP in a complicated health system is a challenge. It requires considering the multiple interlinked factors and elements that individually and collectively influence the adoption and diffusion

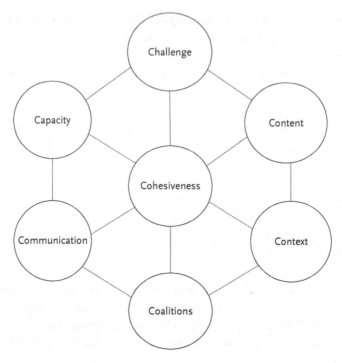

Figure 8.1 The 7 Cs of change.

process. We use a proprietary framework, the 7Cs model, to group these factors into categories. This framework will help clarify the many interconnected elements that will influence the execution of an SIP and hence organize the interventions that are needed. The 7Cs model shown in Figure 8.1 encompasses (i) challenge, (ii) content, (iii) context, (iv) coalitions, (v) communication, (vi) capacity, and (vii) cohesiveness.

The Challenge

Challenge relates to the perception of urgency, severity, scope of threat or opportunity, and importance of the problem or issue being addressed by the SIP. It asks the questions, Why? And Why now? The perceptions around the nature of the problem (e.g., those held by the general public, policymakers, health professionals, and payers) and the narrative around it influence the speed and extent of adoption and diffusion of an innovation, plan, or policy designed to address it.

With more intense challenges, there is greater motivation for change. Challenges that are perceived to be urgent, with large-scale socioeconomic consequences (e.g., the COVID-19 pandemic), typically attract more attention and are looked upon more favorably by stakeholders as an issue that needs addressing.

A crisis can be wasted, however, if leadership is wanting or there is no vision of the change that is needed. Without a vision and plan for change, the momentum created by an urgent challenge will dissipate (Figure 8.2). High-quality leadership is a facilitating factor for implementing change. Without leadership to articulate the need and create concerted action, the change is highly likely to fragment and fail to grow. The attributes of good leadership include clear and inspiring communication, the capacity to arouse trust, and relentless focus on getting results.

The leaders must effectively communicate the reason for change, why the change needs to happen now, what the change will entail, how the change will be introduced, who will benefit and how, and who will be involved in the change process. Undoubtedly, there will be different views on the content and the process of change given the differing values of stakeholders, and conflicts may arise. The leaders need to engage actively with stakeholders to understand when, why, and how these differences arise and work to ensure alignment.

Examples of this kind of leadership facilitating change in the presence of crisis are readily available. The response to the HIV pandemic is commonly cited. At the end of the 1992, HIV infections and AIDS deaths were rapidly rising in low- and middle-income countries and especially in sub-Saharan Africa. The unaffordability of medicines in these countries constituted a clear global crisis among the affected populations.

The leadership response was outstanding. The inspiring leadership of the UN Secretary General Kofi Annan, then followed by South African president Nelson Mandela, the leaders of the Group of 7 countries, and strong leadership of civil society and affected communities, helped to convene the first United Nations (UN) meeting focused on a

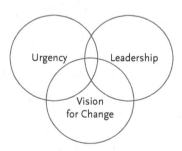

Figure 8.2 Activating a challenge.

disease—HIV/AIDS. Heads of state and representatives of governments met in June 2001 at the UN General Assembly in New York in a special session to discuss the global response to the HIV/AIDS pandemic. At this historic meeting, the heads of state and representatives of governments issued the Declaration of Commitment on HIV/AIDS. They pledged to reverse the epidemic by working collectively with others in international and regional partnerships and soliciting the support of civil society. This meeting had strong support from famous public figures and citizens globally.

The meeting led to a new vision for a global response. The Global Fund to Fight AIDS, Tuberculosis, and Malaria was established to fund the response. The UN coordinated its agencies with the international response, working with inclusive coalitions in countries. These were major changes not just to the global health architecture, governance, financing, and coordination but also to country-level health systems. The initiative established inclusive institutions that brought together state actors, civil society, affected communities, the private sector, international development agencies, and nongovernmental organizations to mount a unified response with highly innovative funding and service delivery models.

The Content

Content is the set and type of changes that your SIP will introduce. It asks the following questions: what is the change, how big of a job is it (e.g., the scale of change), and what is the type of the change? Perceived attributes of the SIP, such as its *relative advantage* compared with the status quo or alternatives, *compatibility* with existing practices, *trialability* in different settings to demonstrate how it might work in practice, *observability* of the effects and benefits, and its *complexity* will all influence the speed and extent of uptake and diffusion.[26]

The content also refers to the underlying typology of an SIP. As presented in Chapter 7 of this volume in the schematic adapted from Argyris and Schön[27] (Figure 7.9), there are at least three major classes of systems problems. The one that describes your problem determines the scope of effort and learning needed to implement your SIP. First-order change problems (those within the existing structure and not needing stakeholder changes) need only single-loop learning to solve primarily mechanistic problems. Second-order problems are adaptive challenges; they modify the existing system structure and create an internal tension that requires that people rethink how they interpret and frame their new experience.

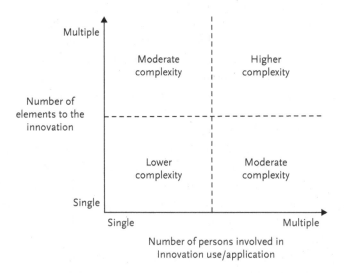

Figure 8.3 Complexity of an innovation.

Double-loop learning is needed for problems that involve these human interactions and values reframing.

The content of the innovation determines its complexity. Complexity of an innovation is the measure of how many different parts or actions an SIP has (Figure 8.3). Complexity is shaped by the quantity of elements in the SIP, the number of stakeholders affected by its application, its frequency of use, and the temporal relationship between its application and effect. Innovations such as the introduction of a new vaccine, a diagnostic test, or short-course medicines are of low complexity, have few facets, and involve limited numbers of stakeholders. Results are rapidly and visibly achieved, and thus readily lend themselves to standardization and replication to reach scale. By contrast, more complex innovations or plans, such as those aimed at changing risky behavior or developing new care delivery models for chronic disease management, involve multiple factors, include many more stakeholders over long time periods, and require greater customization to meet specific needs of different health systems and contexts.

Context

The context refers to the broad contextual factors that influence stakeholder views on the sustainability or need for change of the health system. These include factors such as the demographic and epidemiological transitions, political environment, economic situation, the legal and institutional milieu, technology uptake, prevailing sociocultural norms and practices, culture, and shared societal values, both generally and in the health system where the SIP is being introduced. These factors collectively interact with and influence the health system to create a receptive or nonreceptive context to the introduction, uptake, and diffusion of any innovation, plan, or policy.

The category of culture is vital to understand. We consider culture to comprise two separable attributes for the planner. Where subcategorized under context, culture refers to the anthropologic view comprising the biologic traits, customary beliefs, and social forms of different subgroupings of people, which influence their compatibility with the proposed SIP changes. Different cultural subgroups often have different views of the world. Their folkways reflect their beliefs on important aspects of life— what is good and what is evil, why people get sick, expectations of some types of treatments (like believing that an injection is more powerful than medications taken by mouth), and the meaning of death. We included this type of culture in the analysis of context in Chapter 2 of this volume. Understanding these positions is important because each cultural sector may require unique communication and implementation strategies that fit their beliefs and folkways.

The second type of culture is social. It comprises the shared values, attitudes, and mental frameworks that a nation and its subgroups have adopted. This type of cultural expression is reflected in the distinction we made in Chapter 7 between individualistic and communitarian societies. We come back to this later, when we discuss cohesiveness.

Coalitions

Coalitions are groupings of individuals or parties with a common interest and purpose. Coalitions are critical when introducing a new plan or policy. Coalitions may increase the possibility of uptake and diffusion of an innovation. Identifying and effectively managing opposing coalitions will mitigate the risk of failure.

Coalitions share preferences for joint action. Whether formed to support or oppose an SIP, coalitions are important forces with the potential to help or hinder. Facilitating the development of, and effectively engaging supportive coalitions will increase the possibility of uptake and diffusion of an SIP. Identifying and effectively managing opposing coalitions will mitigate the risk of failure.

Coalitions can be intra- or extra-organizational. Empirical evidence shows that diffusion of innovations in many organizational settings is influenced by coalitions formed by social construction.[28] These include social and professional networks, which are powerful sources of influence and competitive pressures to imitate and legitimize practices,[29] make economic choices,[30-32] and influence political issues. These social pressures might influence positions taken among decision makers,[33] responses to regulatory pressures and institutionalization,[34] the emergence of institutional entrepreneurs,[35] and impact of policy networks.[36]

In the larger societal system, coalitions come in many forms. You should seek to identify coalitions relevant to the adoption of your SIP; they comprise stakeholders affected by or interested in the proposed change. For example, separate or overlapping coalitions in a health system might exist or be formed of insurers, patients, citizens, or politicians, among or between disease-specific, special interest groups, hospitals, or doctors.

The building blocks of coalitions are stakeholders. Coalitions emerge from the interaction and grouping of stakeholders, who are individuals, groups, or organizations affected by an innovation, plan, or policy. Identifying coalitions and their influence requires an analysis of stakeholders (Figure 8.4).

There are six steps in identifying stakeholders and engaging them to form or manage a coalition. The first step involves identifying the stakeholders through a deliberative process to ascertain which individuals, groups or organizations might be in the area of influence from your SIP. The second step involves an assessment of the nature or level of their group's interest, for example high, medium or low. It is important to understand why and how much a stakeholder is interested in the SIP. The third step involves an estimation of the level of influence a particular stakeholder coalition group may have in relation to the adoption and diffusion of your SIP. The fourth step is assessing the direction and level of alignment of the proposed change with each stakeholder grouping, to establish who is supportive and to what extent (e.g., high, medium, or low), and who is opposed. These steps enable a planner to identify possible supportive coalitions that could be formed or identify already formed groups whose resistance to change must be managed. The fifth step involves putting the analysis from Steps 1 to 4 into a single table to create a positioning map of stakeholders (Figure 8.5).

The sixth step of stakeholder analysis and establishment of coalitions is to develop an engagement strategy for the stakeholders. The objective is to consider how supportive coalitions could be developed, as well as how the negative influence of opposing coalitions can be mitigated. Typically, more

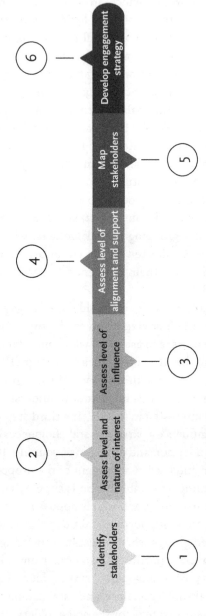

Figure 8.4 Steps in identifying and managing stakeholders.

1 Identify stakeholders

2 Assess level and nature of interest

3 Assess level of influence

4 Assess level of alignment and support

5 Map stakeholders

6 Develop engagement strategy

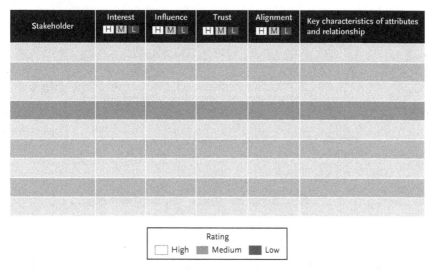

Stakeholder	Interest H M L	Influence H M L	Trust H M L	Alignment H M L	Key characteristics of attributes and relationship

Rating
☐ High ▨ Medium ■ Low

Figure 8.5 Positioning map of stakeholders.

complex innovations, plans, or policies that involve numerous stakeholders at multiple levels in the health system require more intensive stakeholder engagement to establish and sustain supportive coalitions or minimize the effects of hostile groups.

Several general strategies for supporting stakeholders can be pursued depending on the level of interest and support. With a solid understanding of the position of individuals and stakeholder groups, the planner is prepared for careful deliberation about the activities in relation to each stakeholder. In Figure 8.6, we present a simple scheme for making decisions about how to approach developing strategies to manage supportive stakeholders.

For stakeholders who might be opposed to the SIP, a different set of strategies could be pursued (Figure 8.7).

Managing coalitions as individually distinct from one another is a necessary but not sufficient approach to implementation. Inter-stakeholder group alignment and links is an important pathway for building momentum for adoption and diffusion. Coalitions in developed countries fall into two loose groupings—economic and social.[37] Linkages across these interests and vertical nesting of influence groups between local and government levels are powerful enablers of change.[38] Differing values and mental maps often create conflicts that impede change. This will be addressed later when we discuss cohesiveness.

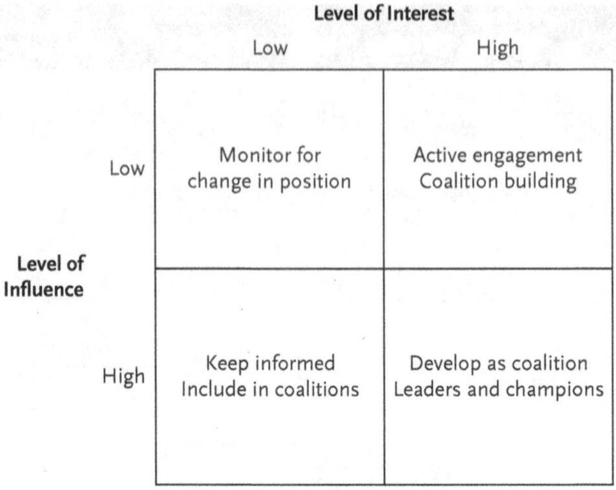

Level of Interest

	Low	High
Low	Monitor for change in position	Active engagement Coalition building
High	Keep informed Include in coalitions	Develop as coalition Leaders and champions

Level of Influence

Figure 8.6 Strategy formulation for developing and managing supportive stakeholder groups.

Finally, differences in attitudes toward risk-taking divide populations into distinctive subgroups or behavioral coalitions of those encountering and considering change. Everett Rogers,[39] in his study of the implementation of government policies targeting farmers, discovered that diffusion was not smooth and continuous. Rather, a group of *early adopters* were attracted to trying out a new practice and readily willing to change. They were the first cohort to adopt the new ideas. Identifying and targeting the

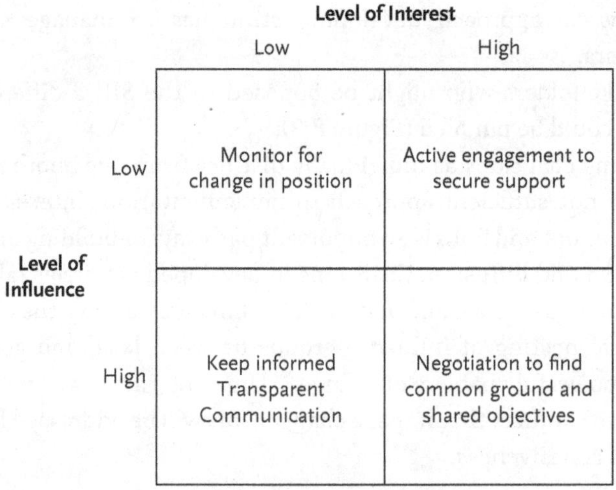

Level of Interest

	Low	High
Low	Monitor for change in position	Active engagement to secure support
High	Keep informed Transparent Communication	Negotiation to find common ground and shared objectives

Level of Influence

Figure 8.7 Strategies for managing opposing stakeholders.

early adopter segment of your SIP audience for your first steps is essential. A second group, called *middle adopters*, was critically important to successful diffusion. This group was skeptical of the change but open to evidence and the experiences of others. Successful implementation depended on the opinions of the early adopters to convince the middle adopters to join in. Bridging the difference between these two behavioral coalitions is often referred to as *crossing the chasm*. A contrasting third group, which Rogers identified as *resisters*, was unyielding and never convinced to change. This group hindered adoption and scale-up of innovations, and their objective was to maintain the *status quo*.

Communication

Communication, the fifth step in the 7Cs model, is essential to explain, promote, and persuade people to adopt your SIP. Communication channels are diverse and audiences vary in their attraction to different modes of learning and listening. Age, culture, education, and socioeconomic factors all influence choice of media. Some prefer newspapers and national news summaries while others are informed via social media. Some communicate informally through social networks while others depend on formal communication such as magazines, newspapers, or religious services.

Regardless of the media used, skilled communication is essential. Regular, clear, and consistent messaging is necessary to promote the challenge (problem) being addressed. Communication should include a persuasive narrative to identify the scope and urgency of the challenge being addressed, identify the benefits of the proposed change, name who will benefit, and articulate what success will look like. It should explain the reason why the change is being introduced now and why the context is supportive for such a change. The target audiences will want to know what is novel and what will change (the content), who will be involved in the change (including the coalitions that will engage and support the implementation process), and how communication will happen (the regularity and source of communication of the implementation process, early tactical wins, and successful outcomes).

The larger the change, the greater is the importance of excellent or extraordinary communication. All too often change programs do not achieve their goals and objectives, because (i) there is no clear narrative to justify the change; (ii) the benefits or targets are not clearly set or communicated to specific target audiences; (iii) stakeholders are not clearly identified or engaged to develop a "winning" coalition supporting change; (iv) messages are not repeatedly reinforced over time; (v) there is no sense of ambition or urgency so that people revert to business as usual; (vi) there are no early tactical wins to gain legitimacy and broad support for the strategic change; (vii), there is no theory of change so that change is rushed and poorly understood,; and (viii) there are no established routines to measure, assess, and communicate progress so that change gets overtaken by other events.

Capacity

The capacity of the health system is the presence or absence of assets and strengths that are necessary to enable the SIP to achieve its proposed results. Successful implementation depends on adequate human, institutional, and financial capacity. Instrumental capacities are predominantly located among the input functions identified in the basic system model in Chapter 2 of this volume. These functions are organization and governance, financing, and resource management. An important aspect of governance is to ensure inclusion, engagement, and social cohesiveness. Separately or linked, leading or supporting change, these functions are the primary leverage points in system transformation and usually the first variables that need to be activated and aligned to support the plan and its implementation.

The capacity of a country to modify its health system is greatly dependent on its ability to adapt and employ these core functions in support of change. One model conceives of the functions as the point of the spear in the change intervention. Here a change in funding, allocation, or governance could itself, or in combination, be the design intervention in the SIP. Alternatively, the improvement could be located elsewhere in the country's system model, in which case the functions would play a key supportive role in supporting and providing the resources and process support to enable implementation of the SIP.

Specific elements in the capacity category can block or facilitate implementation. The functions you identified are givens in your selected health system's status quo. They can either be strengths supporting change or deficiencies that need to be overcome for change to happen. The strengths and weaknesses section of your strengths and weakness, opportunities and threats analysis in Chapter 4 of this volume has already identified some assets and concerns about capacity for change. To the extent possible, your SIP will be helped if it plays to your system's strengths and avoids its weaknesses. In many if not most system changes, there will be capacity shortcomings that will need to be bolstered. These should be identified and remediating plans initiated early.

Cohesiveness

Cohesiveness is a measure of social alignment of stakeholders in a health system. We use the term *cohesiveness* to examine values, mental maps, attitudes, and theories-in-action, and we examine how these influences on different sectors of your target audience will support or impede your SIP. Cohesiveness is the critical ingredient of successful change and sustainability of the system.

We use cohesiveness in two ways: now, as a baseline characteristic before starting, as well as during the process when responses to implementation arise. In the first perspective, cohesiveness is a measure of a country's social solidarity regarding its theory-in-action about how the country works best. Figure 8.8 is a framework to assess where your country stands now on the dimension of individualism versus communitarianism. Broadly speaking, individualistic countries believe they do the best when individuals or stakeholder groups look out for themselves. In very communitarian countries, citizens are aligned in their view that the entire population should share in the benefits from its national enterprise. Each belief has strengths and weaknesses regarding health system function and redesign, and most countries have a mix of these perspectives that inform their shared values. Try picking the spot in the continuum that best describes your country's collective view and position. Consider how its status will influence the adoption and diffusion of your SIP.

The second way to think about cohesiveness is as a measure reflecting the type and level of support generated during the implementation of your health system improvement plan. Most plans for change will generate reactions of resistance or support. Managing those is an important component of that plan's successful implementation.

Cohesiveness marks the degree of national solidarity of views about the health system: what it is, what it does, and how it works. One way to think

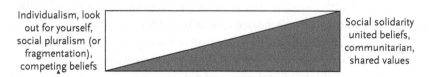

Individualism, look out for yourself, social pluralism (or fragmentation), competing beliefs — Social solidarity united beliefs, communitarian, shared values

Figure 8.8 National status of societal social integration.

about cohesiveness is that it rises when theories-in-use of its stakeholders are aligned with national shared values. Another way to consider this factor reflects the ability of a population to align, or accept and live with differences in interests, attitudes, beliefs, values, and motives among and between health system stakeholders and coalitions. Cohesive populations explore differences. They undertake to understand, resolve conflict between, bridge divergences of, and may even come to agree with conflicting values and beliefs between themselves and others.

Cohesiveness, or its absence, is a major influence on the success of health system interventions. Disagreement and misunderstanding of attitudes, beliefs, values, and motives of stakeholders are major inhibitors of the ability to change. When cohesiveness of stakeholders is high, momentum for change will be enhanced. If the change challenges beliefs of some participants, bringing those views closer in line with others will increase the chances of successful introduction of a change.

We have put cohesiveness at the center of the 7Cs model. It affects all the other elements contributing to implementation. It is important because it is a leading determinant of adoption and diffusion of innovation. Change is facilitated when system problems involve people in the solution and when social interactions are features of the solution. We put shared values and cohesiveness in a category distinct from culture. The latter is relatively fixed; shared values can be a learned behavior.

Cohesiveness and progress in coalescing around shared values are essential elements in successful social change. Because health is one of the most human of all enterprises, most high-impact interventions in health systems encounter social conflict reflecting differences in the way people frame, perceive, and interpret change. The highest impact, highest yield SIP changes are those most likely to encounter disabling, hidden, sealed over, and nondiscussable differences in values, mental maps, and theories-in-use among stakeholders.

The category of the problem an SIP addresses influences how important cohesiveness is to the implementation process. Earlier in this chapter when we discussed content, we alluded to the schema (Figure 7.9) of the three categories of health system problems: mechanistic (first-order change), social (second-order change), and conceptual. Of the three, those involving social relationships are the type of SIP most needing double-loop learning interventions to enhance cohesiveness and facilitate adoption. Second-order health systems problems are likely to involve the type of social relationships that are critical to determining the success of the change being introduced.

Resolving conflicts of interests and values is no easy task. Employing high cohesiveness solutions to work out differences may be the best solution for implementing an SIP with social elements, but it is also the hardest. Double-loop learning, one of the most important tools for managing social change, requires active, often uncomfortable inquiry. The learning involves understanding others' and one's own interests, biases, and theories of how things work and mental frameworks about what is fair or not. Enhancing cohesiveness is no easy process and probably should be reserved for SIPs aspiring to high-impact change. This double-loop learning class of system problem shows up as conflicts between different people's theories-in-action coupled with an inability to discuss them. Underlying disagreements are one of the major reasons why change efforts fail, so it is important to identify these during your planning as potential problem areas to be addressed.

There are several tools to help identify incipient conflict. The first is the 5 Whys, which is a way to dig deeper into the participants' underlying frame and figure out the way they see things. Another good question to ask yourself is, "What must be true for them to act this way." There may be unstated disagreement between groups about the way they understand what's happening, inconsistencies within a single person's theory of how they are behaving and their demonstrable behavior, disabling assumptions and inferences about the actions of others (they are bad; I am good), and cover-ups of the presence of these conflicts, sealing them over and making them nondiscussable.

Four tools are commonly recommended to enhance cohesiveness. They are (i) collaboration, (ii) inquiry and understanding, (iii) communication linkages across stakeholder silos, and (iv) transparency and participation. They are not mutually exclusive and, in fact, probably work best when used in tandem.

First, collaborative engagement is a frequently employed mode of conflict resolution. Cohesiveness is facilitated by effective resolution of conflict. Intense collaborative interactions help stakeholder groups understand others stated disagreements and jointly work to find solutions. Figure 8.9 presents a schematic proposing five different change process approaches to managing conflict encountered while implementing a change.

This schema revisits the model of alternative benefits that citizens value, as presented in Chapter 7. The two axes describe contrasting societal orientations motivating change—economic value-driven and social cohesiveness-driven. This framework is frequently cited in analyses of business leadership approaches to change management.[40] An economic value orientation is one in which the mental map and theory-in-action in use are based on the belief that individuals, organizations, and societies operate best when they are motivated by extrinsic rewards and incentives

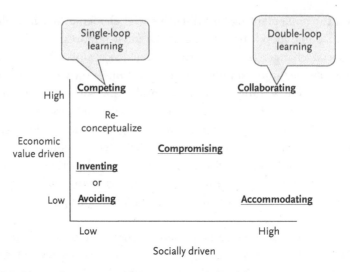

Figure 8.9 System change process drivers: prototypes/models.

such as money, influence, and power. Society is seen as driven forward best by individuals working in their own interest. Rewards and incentives tend to be financial, and status is conferred by the things you own. The United States is most often the example given of this category.

A socially driven society is built on the belief that success depends on a theory-in-action that people are intrinsically motivated and that, once physiologic needs are satisfied, their motivational need is for love and belonging, esteem, and self-actualization. This theory has been popularized in Maslow's concept of hierarchy of needs. In these societies, the desire for social cohesiveness is high. The well-being of the entire community is important. Equity, fairness, and justice are highly desired. The Scandinavian countries are often cited as examples.

Collaboration is a high-effort model best reserved for problems in the double-loop learning category in Figure 8.4. Single-loop learning problems are instrumental and low in social interaction. The solutions for problems low in social interactions are those that energize the animal spirits—competition, problem expertise, focus, intensity, and speed.

You will notice that there are three remaining management style categories—avoiding, compromising, and accommodating. These are commonly in use by those within stable or declining systems. Each is a way of minimizing conflict and effort when a system doesn't perceive a strong need to change but rather is just trying to carry on. Some good health systems with sound strategies are content to avoid rocking the boat—those running successfully in a favorably disposed environment and those nearing the end of a successful period and wanting to save up resources for a later change (a so-called cash cow). And, of course, there are weakening or declining systems that avoid change out of incapacity, unawareness, or fear.

The most popular model for collaborative engagement is presented in William et al.'s book *Getting to Yes*.[41] In it, the authors lay out a series of steps to facilitate productive discussion and resolution of conflict. The heart of their approach is deep understanding of the interests of the competing party and collaborative creation of ideas for solution for both parties—in other words, planning together to get to the best position possible.

The second tool is the aforementioned double-loop learning. It uses a mode of deeply thoughtful inquiry as the basis of learning. Reflective listening opens the possibility of deep understanding of the root causes of espoused positions and views. Reflective inquiry is expressed as being at the heart of the model of double loop learning described by Schön and Argyris in their influential book *Organizational Learning II* published in 1996.[27] In it, the authors describe the theory behind their systems model and give examples of its use in organizations. The double-loop learning model is an approach that exposes and teaches participants to reduce their self-blinding biases, dependence on flawed and undiscussable assumptions and inferences about others, and their use of unexamined theories-of-actions by themselves and others. Better understanding of our hidden biases is, in Schön and Argyris's view, the path to successful resolution of problems and greater cohesiveness.

Third, communication and cross-linking of functions help overcome system siloes and territorial hostility. This approach, built on the life's work of economist and Nobel laureate Elinor Ostrum,[38] emphasizes enhancing and improving interactions among and between disparate groups with overlapping interests, functions, responsibilities, and authority. This approach calls for a polycentric strategy linking vertical authority structures, horizontal interest groupings, and formal operating divisions between social and economic enterprises within society. The process of formally linking, nesting, coordinating, and communicating leads to greater coherence and enhances cohesiveness.

The final tool is to open up the process. Transparency and openness to full participation create the foundation for acceptance of change. When the process is seen by those affected as rational, fair, and open to participation and input from differing perspectives, they are more likely to agree with the conclusions and believe them to be fair and justified. Cohesiveness increases when these criteria are met. Sabin and Daniels,[42] in their book *Setting Limits Fairly*, explore this issue and conclude that accountability, legitimacy, and fairness must be built into the decision processes. In this model, outcomes might differ explicitly, but the process for deciding must be transparent and deemed fair and equitable by the public and, hopefully, the patient affected by the change.

Cohesiveness through social processes is not the only route to adoption of important but controversial SIPs. There are two other often-used ways to reduce intrasystem conflicts and destructive archetypes: these are regulatory rules and market solutions. Each of them has been used to manage system conflict, and both have consequences.

Regulatory solutions are blunt instruments of change that prescribe rules to control behaviors. These interventions may be effective but often leave stakeholders angry and dissatisfied. Regulations often feel unfair or unjust. They emanate from the top levels of government and often merely bury the underlying conflicts, which remain untouched. The result is often that leaders of necessary but unpopular top–down regulatory interventions do so at political risk and suffer electoral consequences. Regulation often leads to an unstable change.

Market mechanisms are a second means to decrease clashes and divergences. Market competition gives individuals more freedom to choose what they want, but the consequences are inequality of access, failure to deliver care where it is needed, and diminished belief in the ideal of medical care as a right.

Of the three interventions to solve resistance to change, social processes to enhance cohesiveness are the most idealistically attractive. Nevertheless, high cohesiveness is open to the criticism that the process of shifting values is utopian. Even if it were associated with the highest adoption and diffusion of an SIP, the pursuit of cohesiveness is best reserved for the category of high-effort, high-impact change.

FORMULATING A CAMPAIGN PLAN

A campaign is a series of connected actions designed to bring about a particular result. A campaign plan is an explicit statement of actions and their timing—in essence an ensemble of activities custom-fitted to your country and your SIP. It answers questions such as what, why, so what, when, where, who, and how? The plan is a roadmap of assembled actions needed to drive your SIP to a successful outcome. It identifies the objective that you need to get to and displays the route you propose to deliver your vision and goals.

The campaign for any health system change is a unique ensemble of activities. There is no one-size-fits-all. Your plan reflects the choices you make to maximize the chances of success. It reflects an understanding of the context and capacity of your health system and country. It taps into opportunities and threats to create urgency and momentum. To get started, the plan specifies the time, place, and first coalitions of early adopters, and it charts the steps in the campaign as conceived at the outset. It identifies what is needed and specifies what is critical.

The 7Cs categories help identify influences that enable a planner to create a country-specific mix of interacting facilitating or blocking factors that your SIP should attempt to address. Consideration of each of the 7Cs stimulates ideas for activities, initiatives, and adjustments to contribute to a plan that is custom designed for your country and SIP. Each of a country's 7Cs categories of influence has strengths to be tapped into and weaknesses to be minimized or avoided.

But a campaign is not simply a matter of addressing all the 7Cs categories. One cannot possibly address every potential influence nor anticipate all emergent problems. A good implementation plan must make choices about its activities. It attempts to achieve the most change possible within the range of facilitating and constraining factors the planners face.

A force field analysis can help make the choices and trade-offs needed to build a strong campaign to implement your SIP. As an example, Figure 8.10 demonstrates how a force field analysis can help identify the opportunities, weaknesses, timing, location, and strength of influences each of the 7Cs. By charting the facilitating and threatening factors for each of the 7Cs, the planner can survey the overall change environment. That high-level perspective makes it possible to identify and select those activities and the sequencing most useful in supporting implementation. The same process can reveal the weaknesses and threats that have the capacity to disable progress. Knowing these enables the planner to create and use the right plan, process, and tools to design a customized campaign.

Implementation of your SIP and its associated changes takes time to introduce and sustain. But while planning is important, all too often too much effort can be spent in planning and not enough on the implementation process itself. Success is determined as much, if not more, by recognizing and adjusting to actual successes and failures as by a beautifully constructed plan. Therefore, the resources allocated for planning and implementation should be used to favor action.

Using the 7Cs Model to Plan the Implementation of Your SIP

In your groups you will now develop an implementation plan. Working independently and following up with discussion in a small group meeting, you should develop an implementation strategy using the 7Cs model.

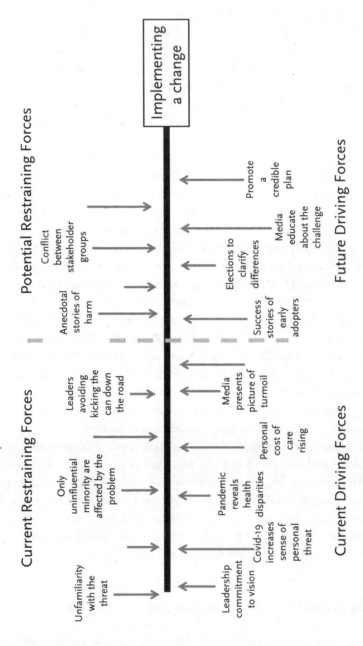

Figure 8.10 7Cs force field analysis using *challenge* as an example.

Frequently, even well-conceived and the best laid out plans are not effectively implemented in practice. This is because the important questions are not posed or systematically addressed. There are seven important questions to consider in relation to the elements of the 7Cs model, each corresponding to an element, and one additional question on the timeline for the implementation. The final step is to put together an implementation plan for presentation and discussion in your country small group meeting.

1. *The challenge: Why is there a need to change?* Where are we going and why are we going there? Explain the sense of urgency to address the challenge now. Identify the challenge that will be addressed by the SIP. Quantify the magnitude of the change. State why it is important to address this challenge and what will happen if it is not addressed.

2. *The content: What should change?* Clearly identify three to five major elements of the SIP and formulate them so that they are understandable to citizens. Identify and describe the targets that must be achieved to reach each major element. These targets should use the SMART schema (simple, measurable, achievable, realistic, and time-bound). The targets should strive to balance visible short-term tactical wins and longer-term strategic outcomes. The former wins support and legitimacy for the SIP and the latter keeps focus on the future changes being introduced that will deliver clear benefits that will accrue to stakeholders.

3. *The context: Why now?* Identify why the SIP should be introduced now. Make a case for the receptivity of the country's context for change. What contextual factors may enable the implementation of the SIP, and what may hinder it? Consider these and set out how you will build on the enabling factors and overcome barriers. In particular, consider how you plan to incorporate contextual issues that can aid or impede the implementation of the SIP.

4. *Coalitions: Who will be involved in the implementation of the SIP?* Formulate who will be involved in the implementation of the SIP and how they will be managed. Identify the stakeholders who will need to be actively managed in the implementation process. Present a stakeholder map by locating each supporting major stakeholders in the 2 x 2 matrix shown in Figure 8.6 and each major opposing (Figure 8.7) and indicate which quadrant they should transition to and your strategy for managing this transition.

5. *Communication: In what way will you communicate about how the implementation will be managed?* How will you inform stakeholders, citizens, and decision-makers about the plan? What are the key messages

and how best would they be delivered? Identify how the SIP will be implemented and what will be achieved. Who will lead? Who is responsible and accountable for the successful implementation of the SIP? Who will benefit? How? Considering the barriers and enablers, the challenge being addressed, and the content of your SIP, articulate your theory of change—presenting how your plan will help achieve the outcomes and how barriers will be addressed.

6. *Capacity: What are the critical organizational, political, managerial, and financial commitments needed for implementation?* Update the health system strength and weakness analysis you first created in Chapter 4 of this volume to remind yourself of your country's capacity levels in relation to the health system functions of organization and governance, financing, and resource management. What are the health system's strengths to facilitate change? What are the weaknesses? What capacities are needed to harness strengths and address weaknesses?

7. *Cohesiveness: What should be the shared values that drive cohesiveness?* First think about the starting point of the population in which you will be implementing your SIP. Your implementation strategy should reflect those aspects of shared national values that will support or impede uptake of your plan for change. Describe how you will use areas of alignment of social values to enhance support for your campaign or how you will anticipate and work your implementation around the resistance you expect when cohesiveness around values is low.

    Second, predict the most likely disruptive conflicts in values and attitudes that your implementation is likely to provoke. You will need to manage these clashes in your implementation process. Pick the one that worries you the most and describe how to handle it.

8. *When will change happen?* Achieving change will require building a sense of urgency with an ambitious yet realistic timeline and effort to ensure achievement of milestones and targets. Progress with achievement of milestones and targets should be regularly reviewed and communicated to all members of the team as well as the stakeholders and coalitions, whose ongoing support for the implementation is critical for change and sustainability.

You should develop a plan of action that lays out the sequence of steps that must be taken or the activities that must be performed to achieve the objectives of the SIP. In this plan of action identify the activities that will be undertaken in the first 18 to 24 months. List these activities and display them on a PERT chart or another timeline by the month when they will be implemented and when the proposed target will be achieved. Provide supporting text to identify who will implement the actions and manage the risks.

PRESENTING RESULTS TO SMALL AND LARGE GROUP MEETINGS

Your small group will meet to discuss the plan proposed by each group member. You are expected to spend about 20 minutes on each student's presentation. At the end of this process, the group should discuss and consolidate around one SIP for presentation to all students and faculty. The group should put the elements together in a timeline and prepare a 10- to 15-minute presentation of your group's SIP and implementation plan in the final large group meeting.

Your audience is the leadership (played by your colleagues in the course) of your health system (i.e., key people in your system whom you need to convince to get formal approval for the time, money, materials, and personnel that would be needed to implement your proposal). As you write your implementation plan, think about how well it anticipates the responses to the questions in Box 8.1.

Box 8.1: UNDERSTANDING YOUR AUDIENCE

- What's the likely assessment of the implementation plan you've identified?
- What evidence or data would they want before buying into how your plan manages changes in the delivery system and practice?
- Who else in the system would be involved in making this plan happen?
- On what aspects of the plan might your audience agree or disagree, and how would you need to work together if you were going to implement this plan?

In the final large group meeting, each small group will present their SIP using their story board from Chapter 6 of this volume combined now with their implementation plan and timeline. In this meeting, students will present in their subgroups of three or more. The presentation should treat the full group membership as the audience that this SIP must convince for approval to move forward. Feedback should be given after each presentation. At the end of presentations, the large group should discuss how persuaded they were by the multiple presentations that the SIP should be supported to implement. What did they like? What could have been improved?

Each small group should present their country and SIP together. All storyboards should have some space for voting either by writing or by Post-its®. Each group will have 10 to 15 minutes to present, followed by 5 minutes of reaction, comment, and critique led by a selected first reviewer. If the schedule can be adhered to, three subgroups can present per hour and all the groups can present and vote in a morning or afternoon session.

At the end of the presentations, all students are given three Post-it® notes, which they should separately label a 1, 2, and 3. They should pick the three SIPs most deserving of receiving support to move on to implementation. Their top choice should receive their 3 and so on. After everyone has voted, each small group should meet briefly to assess the results and ask themselves what they could have done better to receive funding to go ahead.

CHAPTER 9

So What? Who Cares?

The Wrap-Up

The greater danger for most of us lies not in setting our aim too high and falling short but in setting our aim too low and achieving our mark.
—Michelangelo

The final question for those learning from this workbook is "So what?". Why is health system redesign worth the effort? One answer is simple. The world has learned much over the past century about the many policies and interventions that can help improve the health of nations, and those that do not. And all nations have experienced the price to be paid —the rising proportion of GDP that healthcare consumes. We need to learn from these lessons. Bringing better health to a defined population at a cost it can afford is an existential issue for health systems.

In this closing chapter, we raise four "So what?" issues that our fellow learners and aspiring health system designers should address:

- getting good value for money while simultaneously satisfying individual consumers of care, guaranteeing that all citizens can access the health care their nation provides, and assuring that healthcare is appropriately balanced with other national priorities;
- understanding the system's stage of development and capitalizing on a zone of opportunity for innovation still available in all existing health system designs;
- comprehending what a reconceptualization of health systems means, understanding when it is important to consider, and giving some examples of what it might look like;

- appreciating that a high-value health system needs to be owned by all and requires that each and every citizen do their part in preserving, protecting, and sustaining it.

IS A HEALTH SYSTEM PRODUCING GOOD VALUE-FOR-MONEY, SATISFYING INDIVIDUAL CONSUMERS OF CARE, AND GUARANTEEING THAT ALL CITIZENS CAN ACCESS CARE?

Health Systems Are Being Challenged in Their Pursuit of Value-for-Money

In Chapter 7, an expanded value-for-money proposition was presented, emphasizing four general objectives that comprise a high-value health system today. A well-designed system should be *effective* at producing health and health services. It should be *efficient* and affordable. A health system should also satisfy its citizens by delivering on a mix of two important expectations—that the system be *equitable*, empathic, and available to all and that it be *empowering*, patient-centered, and personally satisfying in each *individual's* experience of care. The model of health systems in middle- and high-income countries today, as described in Chapter 3 of this volume, is showing signs of strain achieving these objectives. These symptoms are a portent of things to come. Now is the time to intercede.

First, controlling the inexorable rise of healthcare costs is a priority for maintaining sustainability. The obvious initial interventions should seek to reduce inefficiency and wasteful practices by making the existing systems run better. The tools are improved efficiency and effectiveness. These economizing steps are the first priority in defending a health systems' functionality. A better run system buys time and holds off the inimical effects of The Tragedy of the Commons, which will continue to stimulate demand and raise costs, threatening equitability, acceptability, and sustainability.

Second, a high-value system that holds down costs in the future will inevitably need to set limits on some care. A universal healthcare system cannot afford to cover every medical intervention that is possible. Clearly, any system's blueprint for change and improvement should strive for design changes that not only lower cost but increase value by setting limits on low-value care. When a nation implements a design that redirects investments to favor those services that deliver higher value, that change is a winner.

Setting limits in a universal national health service will be painful and unpopular. When low-value care is traded off for services that provide higher value, some citizens will be denied care that they deem to be important. Some useful tests, treatments, and services will be limited for many who now receive them. The mechanisms to do so will differ, but anger and resentment can be expected among those who are affected. The change process must justify that action to users who are upset. How well the system mitigates their anger will determine its ultimate success. This depends on how convinced the population is that their overall health will be maintained or improved and their health services will be made financially sustainable.

Third, reducing costs and limiting provision of low-value services will lessen income for specialist doctors and hospitals. Because this complex care, not all of which is of high value, is where the great majority of health system expenditure goes now, it will be this sector where the biggest relative reductions must take place. Healthcare is such a high proportion of national expenditures that shrinking it will be a drag on the economy. Specialists and hospitals are a powerful political block that will resist change. Nations will need fortitude to withstand these special interest groups, especially because the latter will mobilize allies to block redesign of health systems that threaten their livelihood. It will take strong leaders to win these battles. Leaders will need a credible, clear, and persuasive story to convince the nation that winning this battle will result in better lives in the future and that giving in to continued rising costs will endanger other benefits they now enjoy as a high-income country.

Finally, systems in general are homeostatic—they resist change. Systems seek to maintain the status quo and will push back against change. Every important function and interconnection will react to the threat and send signals back through feedback loops that attempt to nullify or modify the proposed change. Identifying the most vulnerable driving forces of a system will help a planner anticipate how the proposed changes might influence that critical point and make it possible to predict the unintended consequences. With an idea of what to look for, a change agent can monitor for early warning signs that can help them react quickly, attempt to block or correct for adverse outcomes, and test how strong resistance or support will be.

What Elements Are Crucial in Producing a High Value Health System?

In any system, there are critical inflection points that are the major contributors to how the system works and produces its results. These points often represent the best foothold to initiate improvement. Change at an inflection point can accelerate a transformation or, if handled badly in the design, can lead to severe unintended consequences and failure.

It is essential to know which elements to consider as we try to improve our current health system model. Table 9.1 lists our personal compilation of

Table 9.1 A CHECKLIST OF CORE ATTRIBUTES OF A HIGH-VALUE NATIONAL HEALTH SYSTEM

Core Attribute	Description	Effectiveness	Empowerment	Equity	Efficiency/Cost
• First access care	Ensuring the availability of well-trained, accessible, affordable clinicians to provide primary care	++	++	++	++
• Advanced medical care capacity	Building skills, know-how, and infrastructure to enable clinical specialists, technology, and hospitals to manage complex, treatable illness	+	+	0	–
• Social support	Establishing programs to effectively address poverty, frailty, and management of end of life	++	+	+	–
• Triage at the interface of primary and hospital care	Putting in place a process to identify patients' needs and determine for whom complex hospital-based medical care is appropriate	++	–	– –	++
• Equity, health care for all	Providing access to health care for all—based on need and not on ability to pay	++	0	++	–
• Setting goals, and expectations, then allocating resources	Instituting a process whereby a nation allocates its available money among competing needs	+	0	++	+
• Measurement and management	Setting measurable targets and analyzing achievement	+	0	+	+

• Deciding what benefits are to be covered	Establishing a trusted mechanism to evaluate and set priorities about the benefits a health system should provide	++	–	+	++
• Citizens to do their part	Following good health practices and supporting the health system	++	0	0	++
• Prepared work force	Developing well-educated, accredited and empowered health professionals	+	+	+	0
• Public health	Funding population-based interventions to improve health	++	0	+	+
• Targeted health interventions	Building programs for different population groups to improve disability/death from specific conditions	++	0	0	+
• Allowing private top-up	Letting services be available privately for those who can pay	0	++	– –	+
• National scorecard on health'	Instituting mechanisms to enable regular assessment by nations how their system is performing against expectations	+	0	+	+

Abbreviations: – –, strong incentive to reduce; –, moderate incentive to reduce; 0, no clear incentive; +, moderate incentive to increase; ++, strong incentive to increase.

key attributes of today's successful health systems. These are our candidates for 'must-have' functions to construct a high-value system now. This table is a checklist to consider in designing a high-value health system that can produce healthcare services that deliver good health and satisfaction at an affordable and sustainable low cost. Each attribute is described, and its effect on the four high-value goals is explained.

1. *First access care* is important because primary care is the most cost-effective way to give an entire population immediate access to care and a core set of services, with a doctor and health team who know them. Primary care is the most frequent, and often the only, contact with the health system for most of the population. The services that are delivered include advice, diagnosis of illness, a personal relationship, disease prevention, and management of most common problems. A good experience with primary care enhances satisfaction with and popularity of the health system. Primary care is efficient and cost-reducing because of its accessibility and capacity to treat those with common medical problems. Primary care is universally recommended as a core element of healthcare.

2. *Advanced medical care* is expected to be part of the health systems of middle- and high-income countries today. A system that can deliver cost-effective advanced medical care is a requirement for producing high-value, quality results and satisfaction, and it is a source of national pride. The popularity of such a high-tech, rescue-oriented capacity creates the risk that it expands beyond producing effective and appropriate care and becomes a source of wasteful expense without benefits to patients. Because advanced care is the major driver of healthcare costs, these services are a major design target for improvement.

3. *Social supports* are important services in many health systems. As populations in middle- and high-income countries have aged, the needs of elderly, disadvantaged, and disabled citizens have risen. Providing support is not just a call on the moral obligation of a nation but also a major influence on the four high-value goals. Healthcare services are often the backup when social needs go unmet. The availability of social supports for those who need it, it is argued, reduces direct medical care costs.[1] Meeting these social needs effectively and with respect and dignity enhances both personal and national satisfaction.

4. *Triage* at the interface between primary and hospital care is essential to assure appropriate and efficient use of costly advanced medical care. Utilization of the physical and monetary resources of advanced medical care must be carefully managed to produce the most health for a

nation's money. The better that access to advanced care is managed, the sounder the use of the service's capacity and the lower the costs. Establishing who will benefit most from advanced care requires a clinically sophisticated decision process that is viewed as fair by the population. Much of this triage is now carried out by primary care and hospital doctors, although with little transparency or explicit criteria.

5. *Equity* of accessibility to services is widely held as a necessity in today's health system design. Healthcare is almost universally seen as a human right, to be based on need and not ability to pay. And yet healthcare access varies widely, from those countries where it is free-for-all to other nations in which financial or other barriers to care persist. Defining what should be covered and setting limits fairly are critical requirements in operationalizing a nation's commitment to equity.

6. Setting goals and allocate resources accordingly. Healthcare consumes a large proportion of a nation's gross domestic product. Healthcare's draw on budgets represents an opportunity cost and other areas, such as education and environment, may not receive adequate resources. The goals and resources spent on healthcare should assist a nation to be productive and internationally competitive; national productivity sets the limits on a country's resources available for a nation's health system and other services. Setting goals and making and defending allocation decisions that support strategic national goals is evidence of good political leadership.

7. *Measurement and management* are two essentials in understanding and improving performance. Without defined goals and measurable targets, the work product of health professionals cannot be evaluated nor the care process improved. Healthcare has long lagged other economic sectors in defining and assessing what outcomes and benefits it yields. Whether implicitly or explicitly, decisions about healthcare investment are being made; in our own view, it is in the best interests of doctors to be taking the lead in defining and then evaluating their results. Management is essential in optimizing cost and outcomes. A health system must be considered by its users to be competent if trust and pride in the system are to be maintained.

8. *Deciding what benefits* are to be covered is an essential function. No health system can provide everything to everyone, so choices must be made and some benefits will necessarily be excluded from a benefits package. The process of priority-setting should be evidence-based, fair, transparent, and trusted. Many countries create an independent entity to create some distance and detachment from the funders, policymakers, users, and providers.

9. *Citizens should do their part*. Personal health risks such as obesity, physical inactivity, substance abuse, and smoking are the dominant drivers of chronic illnesses, with their attendant high costs of care. These need to be addressed by individuals. Also, a health system should be "owned" by the entire population, and citizens should view themselves as stewards of their system.

10. A *prepared work force* supports all four parts of the value proposition. Provider education, training, infrastructure support, and accountability assure that benefits are effective and efficiently delivered. Satisfaction with personal healthcare services is enhanced by both the perception and reality of good performance.

11. Strengthening *public health* should be a priority. Over the years, public health has suffered from underinvestment in many if not most middle- and higher-income countries. This weakness has been painfully revealed in the Covid-19 pandemic. In terms of value-for-money, public health is a high-priority investment. Many public health initiatives are far more cost-effective than if delivered as individual medical care services. Robust, expanded public health will improve effectiveness and efficiency and expand the capacity of health for all.

12. *Targeted* health interventions for population groups can be high value when appropriate conditions present opportunities. Prevalent and population-specific health problems can often be managed better through targeted programs, improving health and reducing costs. Large gains in national effectiveness can be achieved.

13. Allowing *private top–up* for those willing to pay extra can be an important way to increase individual satisfaction and reduce the costs of the national health system. Private payers must first pay their share of the public system but then may opt out privately if they wish, thus reducing demand. A self-pay option for those who expect more than the public system provides and are willing to pay for it reduces criticism from dissatisfied citizens who could undermine confidence and satisfaction with a tightly run and priority-based system. While a private system theoretically could undermine the sense of equity among citizens, there is little evidence that has happened in countries with strong national healthcare systems such as England and Australia.

14. Creating a *national scorecard* on health has several benefits. It can facilitate a nation-wide feeling of joint ownership and solidarity. Developing a scorecard can facilitate an open priority and goal-setting process. It can enhance public trust. High national system regard is essential to winning political support, enabling the system to offset the demand

for individual services while meeting explicit goals of universality, effectiveness, and sustainability.

The list of attributes in Table 9.1 is relevant to our present model of health systems as they exist today. All middle- and high-income countries work from common basic assumptions about what a health system is and what it should be expected to do. Health systems and the context within which they are situated are not static. They are constantly evolving. There must be continuous innovation and learning to ensure each of the attributes are in place and are improved to create high-value health systems. There are ample opportunities and important reasons to improve current health systems working within our prevailing paradigm. Our basic shared values about healthcare will not change soon. The checklist is a reminder of things that have worked to make health systems better now. As we noted in the last chapter, even working within the paradigm does not mean that populations will understand and agree to changes designed to improve the system. Conflict is inherent in change. Rather, even within the present paradigm, there will still be clashes of interests and values that will entail deep double-loop learning and inquiry to move to a better system.

Health System Design Conflicts and Tradeoffs

In the title of this wrap-up chapter, we asked, "So what? Who cares?" In one simple view, the answer is that health is important and everyone should care deeply. But there is a more sophisticated view that has been presented during the process of learning how to design changes that increase the value of a health system. Systems are sometimes caught in unpopular trade-offs while striving to achieve an optimal balance between the four high-level goals. Leaders cannot avoid these challenges to their national health system. If a nation fails to solve its trade-off problem by improved design, it faces the threat of requests for more funding, encroachment of health on other national priorities, and limitations of benefits. The consequences of inaction are either degradation of the quality and availability of services provided in healthcare delivery or unsustainable draining of a country's national resources across all sectors of public services from education to defense and beyond.

We have little experience of achieving major reductions in healthcare costs and managing trade-offs. No country has a unique formula for success. Nor are countries alike enough to be optimistic about finding one solution to fit all. If ever there was a need for innovative designs to hold on to an effective, acceptable, and affordable system, it is now. This is a time for experimentation, learning and innovation. New models will be needed to find ways to reduce and better allocate the resources expended on health.

What have we learned about design of high-value health systems in the past half century or more that can guide their redesign and improvement? We do know that there are three basic tools available to heighten value production and reduce costs. These are great leadership, regulation, and market forces. Nations differ in their existing capacity to deploy one or more of these tools. Most innovations and improvement will need a mix of all three.

Where great leadership exists, populations can be persuaded to accept trade-offs. They can be inspired to sacrifice for the common good. Entrusted leadership, combined with faith in government, can convince citizens of the importance of preserving access to low-cost, high-value care while limiting nice-to-have services in the interest of sustaining health care for all.

In nations where consumerism and market forces are strong, market interventions can be designed to improve value. For markets to work, the benefits and prices of products must be accurate, clearly available, and equally understood by both supplier and consumer. We are far from that in any population where market forces are used now. This is a major development challenge for those who propose that market forces can increase value in their national health system. Competition and market forces can be a powerful means for allocating resources but using ability to pay as the criterion for access to care is an important risk that most countries have sought to avoid.

Regulation is frequently utilized when priority-setting is needed and can be an important tool in future. Benefit coverage can be regulated and limited. Reductions in what is covered can undermine national acceptability of the health system, however. Moreover, general regulation is a blunt tool that does a poor job at assessing case-by-case need and potential benefit. For this reason, nations have been cautious in their use of explicit criteria of coverage or regulatory rules that govern access to tests or treatments.

Most nations have relied on priority-setting being carried out implicitly and keeping the resulting decisions hidden from public view. The mechanism is that these decisions are made on a case-by-case basis by doctors at the point of referring patients for higher cost tests and care. In England, this decision is informed by a transparent process that involves economic evaluations conducted by the National Institute of Health and

Care Excellence to advise which interventions and services should be available or used in the National Health Service in England. Doctors triage individual patients based on their assessment of need for and benefit of a referral and the available capacity of often-constrained hospital services.

Observations and Lessons Learned about System Design

Here are some observations that we consider to be design truisms:

- If a national health system for all is perceived as good enough, it doesn't have to be perfect or cover everything for it to pass the test of acceptability.
- Good enough is more than just clinical outcomes and overall health; it also includes a satisfying personal experience when service is received as well as a feeling of good will that the system is fair to all;
- A country's population appears willing to consider its national system to be fair and will tolerate the inequity of having top-ups in services available privately for those who have the ability to pay twice—once for the national service to ensure solidarity and additionally for private care.
- Since an increase in expenditures is inevitable, every national health system must find a way to control costs in their public system; the money to be saved is predominantly in secondary and tertiary medical services, which constitute a majority of expenditures.
- The first step in reining in costs is to improve efficiency and effectiveness before reducing services, but these can only go so far in delaying the need to prioritize benefits.
- When benefits and services must be limited, the reductions should target low-value services and maintain or enhance those of high value. The highest value production in health systems is likely to come from restoring and enhancing public health even if it means reducing individual medical care benefits.
- The more satisfying nonclinical service characteristics are, the less dissatisfaction will emerge from constraining clinical benefits.
- We will have to find good ways to define *need* and prioritize care. There are many routes to allocating resources as acceptably as possible. We need to learn how to prioritize in a way that maintains a national sense of fairness and social solidarity. The way to accomplish this will be different for

every country and represents the major area of design innovation and experimentation to support health systems in the future. The process should be transparent and open. Finally, the process of defining need and setting priorities must be viewed by citizens as inherently fair.

- Some of the cost savings will be reallocated to public health, whose importance and urgency for beefing up after years of relative underfunding have become obvious during the Covid-19 pandemic. Other savings should be visibly directed to social determinants of health, such as recovering economically from Covid-19 and protecting the growing number of citizens whose lives are diminished and in danger from deprivation.

LIFE STAGE DEVELOPMENT OF A HEALTH SYSTEM AND THE OPPORTUNITY FOR CHANGE

Health system change, like most things new, is rarely at its design potential out of the box. Inertia, delays, resistance, mistakes, the learning curve, unexpected events, and unintended consequences are all reasons why learning curves look like the one presented in Figure 9.1. With time, effort, and resources, the system improves to the point where it approaches its design limits, value generated by the system levels off, and progress becomes harder to realize.

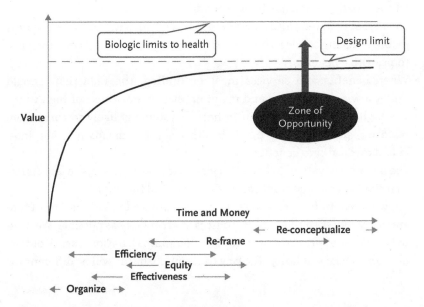

Figure 9.1 A health system developmental life cycle.

Life Stages in Health Systems

There is a progression in the interventions that work at different times during a system's life cycle. Figure 9.1 illustrates a developmental model of health system improvement. In the early stages, organization, effectiveness, and efficiency are the focus of change. Mechanistic problems are a primary challenge; organization is needed just to make the system function at a basic level. Shortly after, however, significant weaknesses and strengths emerge. Efficiency becomes a tool for early system design interventions as waste, rework, duplication, underuse of resources, and lack of coordination become evident. Effectiveness concerns, such as inappropriate tests and treatments, mistaken diagnoses, and poor service present themselves. At this stage equity becomes an important consideration to ensure that different population groups are able to access healthcare services and receive effective care. When the cost of change ultimately encounters declining yields of improvement, transformative change is needed. A change in thinking and reconceptualizing the problem and solutions emerges as a goal and means.

Designers have long worked on increasing health benefits, reducing costs, and satisfying patients. Our current health systems now strive to reach these goals for both individuals and the population as a whole. The tools and approaches fit broadly under the three goals: (i) to improve benefits, we emphasize effectiveness and equity—to deliver the right thing at the right time to the right person or group and in the right way; (ii) to reduce costs, we look to efficiency, thought of simply as doing things right— the goal is to reduce waste and increase productivity; and (iii) to enhance satisfaction, we look especially to fairness, relationships, and improved experience with the services provided.

First priority of the system designer is to fix what doesn't work in the system's structure. Any health system is capable of improving up to the capacity of its design constraints. The structure of medical care delivery in every country is the major determinant of its function. As has been pointed out, the design of a racing car is what determines its performance—how fast it can go and how efficient and reliable it is. Management is what determines the degree to which it can achieve its full design potential. But almost all systems function at levels below their design capability. From the perspective of getting the most health from its investment, a country must optimize its system to produce the most health value for the financial resources it has available to spend.

As presented earlier, the designer balances four value-enhancing performance targets for improvement, which are not mutually exclusive. Broadly speaking, these are efficiency, effectiveness, equity, and consumer empowerment. First priority is to improve the efficiency and effectiveness—doing things right and doing the right things—within the constraints of the design of the system to squeeze the maximum output achievable while keeping down costs, Greater productivity can be accomplished by increasing the efficiency with which services are delivered to the end user. The traditional tools for improving efficiency are identifying errors, slowdowns and backups, and waste and reducing them by controlling variation through tools such as statistical process control methods, lowering the input costs of producing the services through using lower paid, using less trained personnel to deliver the service, shifting more of the services to the patient themselves, and deploying technology that streamlines processes.

Effectiveness in practice means providing more of the right benefits and less of the wrong. The greater the effectiveness of the health system, the higher the value produced by the service. Reducing low-value care while maintaining or adding high-value services is one way to enhance value. To know how we are doing, the system needs to assess objectively the value of the service by measuring its documented beneficial outcomes and costs.

Effectiveness is heightened especially by interventions that improve clinical decision-making and enhance prevention. Many studies demonstrate wide variation and inappropriate diagnosis and treatment by doctors. Much effort has been put into improving doctors' performance, but progress has been slow, and old habits stubborn. Prevention is almost always the most effective way to treat disease. In our existing health systems, prevention to improve health and wellness and delay the development of disease is probably our best option for improving effectiveness. Our experience suggests that delivering prevention through the medical system may not be the optimal method. Population-based, public health interventions might be a more cost-effective model.

Improvement in the category of effectiveness involves doing more when the benefits outweigh their added costs and doing less when the benefits are below the costs to produce them. For example, we can think of individual healthcare as drawing upon a long list of possible interventions. Some have no benefit and should be dropped from funding. Others have limited benefit but may cost a great deal because the intervention is very costly or the intervention is of small benefit but applicable to large numbers of patients. Within that category are many tests and procedures that are done without adequate consideration of the probability of benefit or harm.

The third national value target is equity, to ensure that citizens feel that they have fair access to a set of effective services when they need them. The single most important tool is adequate public funding to provide affordable insurance for those without the resources to pay for care themselves. Delivering healthcare for all regardless of ability to pay is a major source of national satisfaction and solidarity.

The fourth national value target is empowerment—improving responsiveness of health system to meet citizens' personal needs and the experience and satisfaction of individual citizens with their health system. Because some services will inevitably be limited for some people, we can expect individual satisfaction to be under threat in a system that is designed for optimizing national value and affordability. In a well-designed high-value population health system, individual dissatisfaction is mitigated by dispensing services with dignity and respect, maintaining a fair process of deciding what should be available, and inspiring pride and solidarity through fairness and providing services where they do the most good for the most people. If this can be done well, both national and personal satisfaction should be maintained.

Unexplored Zone of Transformative Change

Health systems have an absolute ceiling on the benefits they can deliver no matter how much is spent. Even if a perfect system were able to keep every citizen mentally and physically at the top of their potential for a lifetime, the country still would face the unavoidable biologic constraint of a health system—death, hopefully in old age. And as that inevitable limitation gets closer, the less value a health system is able to produce no matter how one chooses to measure it. Disability inevitably increases and function declines no matter how much a nation tries to avert it. No health system can break through that ceiling.

However, between that outer limit and the maximum value a country produces from their current health system design lies a gap that we have called the zone of opportunity (see Figure 9.1). This zone is open season for system design innovation. When performance is improving in early development and there is much opportunity available to make it better, pressure to break into the zone is low. Eventually, value production encounters growing constraints and the inherent limitations of its system design. The opportunity to enhance value through operational improvements is diminished. The point we are making is that efficiency and effectiveness interventions are most beneficial when the gap between the actual and theoretical design potential of a model is large. Innovation in design in the zone of opportunity is of greatest value when a model has reached close to its maximum design potential. The greatest gains remaining at that point are those created by changing the health system design through reconceptualization and transformative design, as described in the next section.

RECONCEPTUALIZATION AND TRANSFORMATIVE CHANGE IN SYSTEMS DESIGN

We believe that all health systems will ultimately reach the limits of change possible within their current design framework. A system's context is constantly shifting. Technological and scientific innovations, economics, attitude change, and disabling archetypal features like The Tragedy of the Commons will overtake the capacity of first- and second-order change designed from within a system's existing paradigm. The products of the system eventually fail to meet the need generated from the evolution of a system's consuming and supporting environment. Thomas Kuhn, in his book *The Structure of Scientific Revolutions*,[2] describes the difference between incremental change from within a paradigm and transformative breakthroughs possible when a paradigm changes. Our contemporary health system archetype, or paradigm, has been shaping health systems since World War II or before. Within this framework, variations of design are ones we can either know or imagine. Even when innovations are created, they are from within our contemporary mental set; all are based on what we know. If the basic paradigm were to change from that of what we now consider to be successful high-value health systems, the new system would have to identify and develop its own unique attributes.

Our present-day shared paradigm shapes how we view the world of health systems. It is so familiar to us that we are largely unaware how much it influences our views of health care. Experiencing health systems through the existing framework creates a kind of optical delusion (as Einstein said) of truth and permanency and a sense that what we perceive of it today is the only way that health systems can be. This confidence is built from a foundation of long-established mental maps comprising such beliefs as ethics, values, economic views, assumptions about human nature, know-how, expectations, and more.

To break out of the straightjacket of an existing paradigm requires reconceptualization as shown in the problem typology model (see Figure 7.9 in Chapter 7 of this volume). We now present this third way of designing for improvement as a path for a nation to change the rules of the game imposed by their current knowledge, know-how, and mental maps. That is to change the maps themselves.

Two examples (and there surely are others in the arena of health systems change) illustrate past paradigm shifts and help us understand how they were generated and the conditions under which a new paradigm becomes acceptable and transformation-in-action is enabled. One is the radical change involved in starting England's free-at-the-point-of-use National Health Service in the late 1940s and the role of an out-of-the-box thinker in conceptualizing and advocating for a new social welfare state. The second example is a public initiative to lower costs and extend coverage by limiting benefits in the Medicaid (America's insurance for the poor) program in the state of Oregon.

Creating the National Health System in England

Inspired by Franklin Roosevelt's Four Freedom's speech but disappointed in America's ability to heed it, William Beveridge was a leading conceptualizer and persistent advocate for a cradle-to-grave social welfare system for England. He was irritating in pushing his cause but did not care. Judged an irascible, arrogant, opinionated, and brusque academic by contemporary politicians, he was passed over for an operational position in the wartime government by offering him the chairmanship of a commission to study the existing social insurance and make recommendations. He presented a report in 1942 recommending that the government should tackle what he called the "five giants on the road of reconstruction, of Want, Disease, Ignorance, Squalor and Idleness." One of the report's three fundamental goals was to create a national health service of some sort. His report was timely. It was accepted for planning by the wartime government. The postwar Labor government under Clement Atlee passed the general legislation and operationalized the vision for the NHS under the direct guidance of the then–Minister of Health, Aneurin Bevan.

Bevan was a Welsh politician who was appointed a minister in the postwar Labour government. It was his task to operationalize the universal health insurance and design healthcare delivery. His model was the Tredegar Medical Aid Society, a very popular local voluntary insurance scheme in his small Welsh hometown, where townspeople paid a subscription fee to cover the costs of free medical care services. Bevan determined that all medical care should be free to English citizens.

Disappointingly from our perspective as planners of change, the structure of the NHS, which stands intact to this day, was more opportunistic than planned by Bevan. The design grew from a mix of elements including amalgamating a patchy collection of medical practitioners and private and public hospitals. Doctors adamantly opposed the NHS and were determined not to participate. Ultimately, Bevan bought them off by enabling them to remain private and independent. It would be much more satisfying to readers of this workbook if the design had emerged fully articulated in a White Paper. The actual process does illustrate the importance of opportunism and workarounds for implementation if the core vision is held fast.

Little did Bevan realize that allowing a private system alongside the NHS would be a design that would make the NHS better and serve England well. England's public–private mix creates an effective but low-cost, capped public system for all but at the same time enables those who are willing to pay on their own to buy more. We believe that if healthcare is to be affordable for all, most nations will need to move toward such a type of two-tiered system. The first of the two parts will be an affordable basic insurance package that will cover everyone. It will be limited in benefits to those services that are necessary and will be subsidized for those for whom it is still out of reach financially. It will not cover everything that is possible medically and probably will have some caps on expenditures. Consumer choice will be limited, but not absent. It will be a system designed for maximum efficiency and effectiveness but not primarily for choice. But because it is available to all, it satisfies the political requirement of being fair and meets the ethical and moral responsibilities of a nation to provide healthcare for all.

A voluntary private top–up system would be available to supplement the national program. Those opting to use the private system could do so only after having paid their share for the basic system. It enabled those who wish for more, and can afford it, to pay for themselves. In a discretionary private system, consumers can buy what they want; choice reigns. A private top-up system is also where one could test new models of care and figure out how strong consumer choice and market forces could contribute to reining in the growth of costs. Such a private sector also frees up capacity in the public system and removes an articulate but demanding segment of the population. The private opt-out may reduce turmoil and criticism but has the risk that the public system will be under less pressure to improve. As in any consumer market, there are regulatory constraints to protect the consumers in both systems and keep markets working efficiently.

This history illustrates three points about reconceptualization. First, it is more likely to be generated by those outside the existing paradigm of the health system. These innovators are often lone wolves who care little about being mainstream and politically popular. Both Beveridge and Bevan were irritating dissidents within the existing structure. Paradigm change is initially greeted with skepticism and hostility and often is unpopular. It takes someone with a thick skin and an outsider's viewpoint to break from the traditional paradigm.

Second, the history emphasizes the importance of shared values and trust in government. The British suffered mightily during the war and came to the postwar period with a strong sense of national solidarity and great trust in government to work for the betterment of life. This alignment of shared values and collective expectation made the creation of the social welfare state relatively easy.

Finally, perhaps the history of the NHS illustrates the importance of a simple inspiring vision. In Bevan's case, it was that care would be free when it was used. This core belief drove the design of insurance and delivery.

Limiting Benefits in the State of Oregon in the United States

The Oregon Medicaid experiment is an example of an equally radical change but, in this case, limiting rather than increasing benefits. Senator and subsequently Governor Kitzhaber, an emergency doctor, spearheaded an effort starting in 1989 to limit Medicaid benefits (insurance for the poor) so a larger number of recipients would be able to join. Benefits were to be ranked and when the budget ran dry, lower priority services would no longer be covered. The concept was revolutionary.

In fact, the idea was doggedly pursued and ultimately successful. A long list of medical interventions was prioritized, criticized, revised, and ultimately accepted. The process was transparent and accessible. All told, there were 57 public meetings for comment, critique, and suggestions—an extraordinarily open process. In the end, the program became caught up in procedural criticisms from the state's federal partners and was only partially implemented in the form as conceived. The important lesson is that a radical approach to limiting covered benefits was acceptable to the public, through a transparent, open process that was viewed as rational and just.

What Might Radical Improvements Look Like in a New Paradigm?

No one can predict with certainty what reconceptualized health systems might look like in a new paradigm. Nevertheless, unresolvable tensions and conflict undermine the continuation of the way we do things now. Transformative change is alluring. We want to give some examples of transformative potential in our current health systems. In these three examples, existing modes of thinking are already being challenged, creating pressure to change thinking and replace current practice with something fundamentally different.

Example 1: The Promise and the Challenge of Precision Medicine for All

A new paradigm may arise from the growth of precision medicine, which customizes care to address individual genetic variation. Research and development in genetics and genomics are showing that medical interventions can yield clinically significant results by precisely targeting individuals and their diseases (as is emerging with management of conditions such as cancer, dementia, and susceptibility to the complications of Covid-19). These major scientific developments are exciting—benefiting those who are affected by rare conditions. However, the high cost of R&D and commercialization of these new products and small markets (in terms of affected individuals) means the prices for these treatments are in excess of million dollars per person—and not affordable for most countries in the world.

If that trend continues, the existing model of pricing and funding of healthcare is untenable. Affordability of medical care depends on the model that effective medical interventions are applicable to large populations, which thus makes it possible to support the costs of their development and delivery. If it becomes medically important to personalize care to target individual variation in genomes, the user population is reduced, with the current health system financing models R&D costs will be difficult to cover, the costs of treatment will escalate, and the capability of nations to fund such care for all will diminish. If use is limited only to those who can afford to pay privately, the advances will undermine the premise of equitability and care for all. Ultimately, national solidarity will be severely stressed.

Example 2: Exposing the Realities of the Widely Held Belief That Every Life Can Be Saved

Our current systems operate on the assumption that every person deserves care no matter the cost. Our espoused position in middle- and high-income countries is the premise that no effort should be spared to save every life. During the Covid-19 pandemic, Andrew Cuomo, the governor of the U.S. state of New York, in his May 5, 2020 Covid-19 news briefing justified his costly recommendations as follows: "How much is a human life worth? That is the real discussion that no one is admitting, openly or freely. (I believe) that we should. To me, I say the cost of a human life, a human life is priceless. Period." Earlier, he stated, "And if everything we do saves one life, I will be happy."

In fact, this position is a popular and widely held shared belief but clearly unrealistic. It has long been weakened in action in healthcare as elsewhere. Doctors' decisions prioritizing access to healthcare and rationing reflecting social standing and ability to pay have long been present but have largely been nondiscussable in public decision-making. The need to allocate scarce resources, such as intensive care beds and respirators during the Covid-19 epidemic, has begun a process of making the criteria for such decision-making more explicit. Many hospitals around the world have been attempting to develop criteria for whose life may be saved by being enabled to use the limited treatment resources. As conditions such as pandemics, antimicrobial and viral resistance to antibiotics, and complications of chronic illness exceed available capacity, nations will no longer be able to keep allocation decisions hidden. Criteria will be developed to guide who shall receive scarce care. Even though priorities and limits should be set fairly and openly, the very fact of setting limits will force citizens to reframe their belief that each life is priceless and must be saved. In societies that now eschew the idea of agism in healthcare (when older people are discriminated against because of age), a new shared belief about the rights of the elderly will be needed for access to care to be based on the expected years of life gained, suffering reduced or predictions of benefit on the quality and dignity of life.

Example 3: Considering the Risk of Potential Abuse of Medical Technology

The capacity of technology to replace, augment, or manipulate human functions has been expanding beyond imagination. Hardware, either external or implanted, is replacing limbs, regenerating hearing or vision, or preserving communication, as was graphically demonstrated by the technology that enabled astrophysicist Stephen Hawkings to overcome his almost complete paralysis and communicate what he was thinking. In a broader sense, however, medical technology can be seen as any hardware or software that manipulates human development and mental or physical function and behavior. In that interpretation, any intervention can be used to modify our inherited capacity for learning, function, and behavior. Implanted devices, psychedelic and mood-changing drugs, data science, and manipulations of childhood development can theoretically enable us to function better.

Technologies can now alter genetic make-up to improve bodily functions. The same technologies—if they were, let's say, applied preconception to precondition early childhood moral and intellectual development—could also create the personality characteristics Orwell described in his book *1984*.[3] As technology increases its capacity to modify human function, it could easily be abused to create human functionality with adverse consequences—for example, creating military combatants without feelings of remorse for their actions.

The ability of science to modify human function has accelerated beyond our ethical capacity to know how to use it. One of the necessary transformations in how we think about technologic invention is to agree to an enforceable moral framework to manage how we use it.

CITIZEN RESPONSIBILITY IN PRESERVING AND PROTECTING THEIR HEALTH SYSTEM

The final element in transforming health systems is our collective engagement not merely as users and payers but as participant-owners of health systems. The question of "Who cares?" invites two interpretations. These are: who cares *about* their health system and who cares *for* it. All citizens care about their health system. Most have strong feelings about being healthy and high expectations about accessing care at an affordable price. However, few citizens understand the importance to their future of their contributing role in caring for their system. We want to conclude this workbook by stressing the dependence of any health system's survival on the role each citizen plays in caring for it.

An essential goal in design for improvement of health systems is citizen stewardship to make it better and better. As Pogo, a US opossum cartoon character drawn by Walt Kelly many years ago, put it, "we have met the enemy and he is us." The new paradigm for high-value population-based care is that the resource of an excellent, accessible health system must be treated by all as a shared national treasure. In that sense, we argue that health is a resource to be protected by each and every one of us. It is no different than the personal commitment and engagement we recognize as vital to protect our essential physical environment of air, ocean, and land; our common heritage of language and culture preserved in World Heritage Sites like the Taj Mahal; or our sacred beliefs such as the Haj, Easter, Diwali, Vesak, or Yom Kippur, to name several examples.

As citizens, we cannot be passive in our relationship with our health system and expect it to meet our expectations. Until we understand the fragility of our own health system and recognize that our own actions are what is needed to save it, what success we have achieved will continue to be at risk.

Our actions as citizens require first that we take personal responsibility for maintaining health-enhancing habits. Smoking, violence, and eating badly are self-inflicted indiscretions that make us sick and lead to a chronic illness burden that is draining resources from national systems. It isn't adequate to believe that only the transgressing individual suffers. We all pay for ill health, and therefore we have a collective duty to preserve our own health.

Second, patients must activate their own role as essential members of the care team. Healthcare's current expectation of patient behavior is one of passivity. The doctors are in charge. Patients are not held responsible. Patients regress and often accept that others are making the decisions.

In a functional health system, patients can no longer relinquish their active participation when sick. Decisions are being made all the time, and patients need to know the risks and benefits and decide what works for them. When no longer capable of carrying this out, the responsible citizen will have communicated their wishes to those who will be speaking for them.

Third, we must be stewards of the health system. Citizens must be prudent and appropriate in their use of our common resource. We need to learn the rules that improve our health system's efficiency and effectiveness and apply them in our own care-seeking actions. We need to set our expectations to align with the system we have.

Finally, we need to understand the unique limitations in how our health system works. No matter how good a system we have, people will die and survivors will naturally feel that more should have been done. No matter how good a system we have, we must make choices and determine and then actively support priority-setting. The more mature, thoughtful, and engaged a population can be with their health system, the better that system will be in providing equitable accessible for all at a sustainable cost. Participating as though one were a team player in the health system will maximize the health of the nation and create value for all.

CONCLUSION

The next decades will present nations with a sea change in health. Our national health systems have been on a familiar trajectory for the past half century or more, with a generally progressive expansion of benefits and continual increases in the proportion of national resources allocated to medical services. We have consistently raised our expectations about, and our desire for, the heroic accomplishments of medical care. By and large, our citizens have been willing to pay more to access these benefits.

But forces are bringing this growth era to the edge of its end. These include the structural bias of the system archetype of The Tragedy of the Commons. In addition, forces such as the aging of populations, the growth of lifestyle-influenced chronic illness, rising consumer expectations, and growing demand for access to new tests and treatments are stressing the capacity of nations to pay for the additional costs.

Nations have been struggling to find the money to pay for healthcare as the increase in a country's health expenditures have outstripped the pace of national economic growth. This problem will worsen, particularly if global productivity declines and an economic downturn occurs. Paradoxically, the pressure to maintain universal healthcare and existing benefits may actually deter national budgets from expenditures on the nonmedical determinants of health. Climate change, lost jobs, declining income, and stress-induced mental health problems may cause disability and death beyond the capability of medical care to mitigate.

The overall impact of these forces portends fundamental change. Continuing to fund rising costs requires two conditions, neither of which seems likely in the future—the growth of national productivity to increase available financial resources or finding the money for healthcare by taking money from other national government priorities. Medical breakthroughs and efficiency and effectiveness enhancements, valuable though they may be, are not going to increase national productivity by much if at all.

Our goal in this book has been to present an educational approach for others to learn about value-based health care for populations. The premise of the book is that each and every national health system should be striving to maximize the health of its population as efficiently and effectively as possible within the resources a nation decides it can afford and sustain. In this process, we have stressed the importance of the structural design of the health system; design sets the outer limits on performance. However, any system can be redesigned and even transformed in what they produce and how they create value. What is possible for a nation, however, not only depends on its priority health problems but also fundamentally on its values. When fairness, equitability, and responsibility are deep in the shared values of the nation and governments are trusted, countries have abundant design possibilities practically available to improve their health at an affordable cost.

REFERENCES

CHAPTER 1

1. World Health Organization. WHO Constitution. Published April 7, 1948. https://www.who.int/about/who-we-are/constitution

2. Office of Disease Prevention and Health Promotion, US Department of Health and Human Services. Healthy People 2030 Framework. https://www.healthypeople.gov/2020/About-Healthy-People/Development-Healthy-People-2030/Framework

3. Coker RJ, Atun RA, McKee M. Health care system frailties and public health control of communicable disease on the European Union's new eastern border. *Lancet*. 2004;363:1389–1392.

4. Farmer P, Frenk J, Knaul F, et al. Expansion of cancer care and control in countries of low and middle income. *Lancet*. 2010;376:1186–1193.

5. Chen LC. Good health at low cost: from slogan to wicked problem. *Lancet*. 2012;379(9815):509–510.

6. Lavis JN, Røttingen JA, Bosch-Capblanch X, et al. Guidance for evidence-informed policies about health systems: linking guidance development to policy development. *PLOS Med*. 2012;9:e1001186.

7. Evans RG. Incomplete vertical integration: the distinctive structure of the health-care industry. In: Van der Gaag J, Perlman M, eds. *Health, Economics, and Health Economics*. Amsterdam, The Netherlands: North-Holland, 1981.

8. Cassels A. Health sector reform: key issues in less developed countries. *J Int Dev*. 1995;7(3):329–347.

9. Janovsky K, Cassels A. Health policy and systems research: issues, methods, priorities. In: Janovsky K, ed. *Health Policy and Systems Development: An Agenda for Research*. Geneva, Switzerland: World Health Organization; 1996.

10. Anderson G, Hussey PS; Organization for Economic Cooperation and Development. Comparing health system performance in OECD countries. *Health Aff (Millwood)*. 2001;20(3):219–232.

11. Roberts MJ, Hsiao W, Berman P, Reich M. *Getting Health Reform Right*. New York, NY: Oxford University Press; 2004.

12. Murray CJ, Frenk J. A framework for assessing the performance of health systems. *Bull World Health Organ*. 2000;78(6):717–731.

13. World Health Organization. *World Health Report 2000—Health Systems: Improving Performance*. Geneva, Switzerland: World Health Organization; 2000.

14. World Health Organization. *Everybody's Business: Strengthening Health Systems to Improve Health Outcomes*. Geneva, Switzerland: World Health Organization; 2007.

15. Atun RA, Menabde N, Saluvere K, et al. Implementing complex health innovations—primary health care reforms in Estonia: multimethod evaluation. *Health Policy*. 2006;79(1):79–91.

16. Senge PM. *The Fifth Discipline: The Art and Practice of the Learning Organization*. London, UK: Random House Business Books; 1990.

17. Senge PM. *The Fifth Discipline Fieldbook*. London, UK: N. Brealey; 1994.

18. Simon HA. *Models of Bounded Rationality: Empirically Grounded Economic Reason*. Cambridge, MA: MIT Press; 1982.

19. Sterman JD. Learning in and about complex systems. *Syst Dynam Rev*. 1994;10(2–3):291–330.

20. Diehl E, Sterman JD. Effects of feedback complexity on dynamic decision making. *Organ Behav Hum Dec*. 1995;62(2):198–215.

21. Sengupta K, Abdel-Hamid TK. Alternative conceptions of feedback in dynamic decision environments: an experimental investigation. *Manage Sci*. 1993;39(4):411–428.

22. Sterman JD. System dynamics modelling: tools for learning in a complex world. *Calif Manage Rev*. 2001;43(4):8–25.

23. Forrester JW. *Industrial Dynamics*. Cambridge, MA: MIT Press; 1961.

CHAPTER 2

1. World Health Organization. *World Health Report 2000—Health Systems: Improving Performance*. Geneva, Switzerland: World Health Organization; 2000.

2. World Health Organization. *Everybody's Business: Strengthening Health Systems to Improve Health Outcomes*. Geneva, Switzerland: World Health Organization, 2007.

3. Evans RG. Incomplete vertical integration: the distinctive structure of the health-care industry. In: Van der Gaag J, Perlman M, eds. *Health, Economics, and Health Economics*. Amsterdam, the Netherlands: North-Holland; 1981.

4. Janovsky K, Cassels A. Health policy and systems research: issues, methods, priorities. In: Janovsky K, ed. *Health Policy and Systems Development: An Agenda for Research*. Geneva, Switzerland: WHO; 1996.

5. Roberts MJ, Hsiao W, Berman P, Reich M. *Getting Health Reform Right*. New York, NY: Oxford University Press; 2004.

6. Frenk J. Dimensions of health system reform. *Health Policy*. 1994;27(1):19–34.

7. Rifat Atun, Nata Menabde. Health systems and systems thinking. In Cocker R, Atun R, McKee M, eds. *Health Systems and the Challenge of Communicable Disease*. New York, NY: Open University Press; 2008.

8. Senge PM, Kleiner A, Roberts C, Ross R, Smith B. *The Fifth Discipline Fieldbook*. New York, NY: Doubleday; 1994.

9. Senge PM. *The Fifth Discipline: The Art and Practice of the Learning Organization*. London, UK: Random House Business Books; 1990.

10. Sterman JD. System dynamics modelling: tools for learning in a complex world. *Calif Manage Rev*. 2001;43(4):8–25.

11. Samb B, Evans T, Atun R, et al.; WHO Maximizing Positive Synergies Collaborative Group. An assessment of interactions between global health initiatives and country health systems. *Lancet*. 2009;373:2137–2169.

12. Atun RA, Menabde N, Saluvere K, et al. Implementing complex health innovations—primary health care reforms in Estonia: multimethod evaluation. *Health Policy.* 2006;79(1):79–91.
13. Atun R. Health systems, systems thinking and innovation. *Health Policy and Plan.* 2012;27:iv4–iv8.
14. Atun R, Aydin S, Chakraborty S, et al. Universal health coverage in Turkey: enhancement of equity. *Lancet.* 2013;382(9886):65–99.
15. Atun RA, Lebcir MR, McKee M, Habicht J, Coker RJ. Impact of joined-up HIV harm reduction and multidrug resistant tuberculosis control programmes in Estonia: system dynamics simulation model. *Health Policy.* 2007;81:207–217.
16. Atun R, Odorico Monteiro de Andrade L, Almeida G, et al. Health system reform and universal health coverage in Latin America. *Lancet.* 2015;385:1230–1247.
17. Daniels N, Sabin J. Limits to health care: fair procedures, democratic deliberation, and the legitimacy problem for insurers. *Philos Public Aff.* 1997;26:303–350.

CHAPTER 3

1. Organisation for Economic Co-operation and Development. Health Policies and Data. https://www.oecd.org/els/health-systems
2. World Health Organization. WHO Health Systems Database. https://www.who.int/topics
3. Common Wealth Fund. Publications & Data. https://www.commonwealthfund.org/publications-data
4. World Bank. World Development Indicators. https://data.worldbank.org/data-catalog
5. World Happiness Report 2020. https://worldhappiness.report/
6. World Health Organization. WHO Constitution. Published April 7, 1948. https://www.who.int/about/who-we-are/constitution
7. Porter M. *The Competitive Advantage of Nations.* New York, NY: Free Press; 1990.

CHAPTER 4

1. Rawls J. *A Theory of Justice.* Cambridge, MA: Belknap Press/Harvard University Press; 1971.
2. Daniels N. Accountability for reasonableness in developing countries. In: *Just Health: Meeting Health Needs Fairly.* Cambridge, UK: Cambridge University Press; 2007.
3. Schlander M. NICE accountability for reasonableness: a qualitative study of its appraisal of treatments for attention-deficit/hyperactivity disorder (ADHD). *Curr Med Res Opin.* 2007;23(1):207–222.
4. Daniels N, Sabin JE. Accountability for reasonableness: an update. *BMJ.* 2008;337:a1850.
5. Helmer-Hirschberg O. Analysis of the Future: The Delphi Method. Published 1967. https://www.rand.org/pubs/papers/P3558.html
6. Christensen C, Cook S, Hall T. What customers want from your products. *Harvard Business Review.* Published January 16, 2006. https://hbswk.hbs.edu/item/what-customers-want-from-your-products
7. Office of Disease Prevention and Health Promotion, US Department of Health and Human Services. Healthy People 2030 Framework. https://www.healthypeople.gov/2020/About-Healthy-People/Development-Healthy-People-2030/Framework

8. National Health Service. The NHS Constitution. https://www.gov. uk/government/publications/the-nhs-constitution-for-england/ the-nhs-constitution-for-england
9. Madsen D. SWOT analysis: a management fashion perspective. *Int J Bus Res.* 2016;16(1):39–56.

CHAPTER 5

1. Buzan T. *Use Both Sides of Your Brain.* New York, NY: Plume Press; 1991.
2. Washington State Department of Enterprise Services. Root Cause Analysis. https://des.wa.gov/services/risk-management/about-risk-management/ enterprise-risk-management/root-cause-analysis
3. de Bono E. *Lateral Thinking: Creativity Step by Step.* New York, NY: Harper Rowe; 1970.

CHAPTER 6

1. Doran GT. There's a S.M.A.R.T. way to write management's goals and objectives. *Manage Rev.* 1981;70(11):35–36.

CHAPTER 7

1. Sterman JD. Learning from evidence in a complex world. *Am J Public Health.* 2006;96(3):505–514.
2. Roberts C, Ross RB, Kleiner A, Smith BJ, Senge, PM. *The Fifth Discipline Field Book Strategies and Tools for Building a Learning Organization.* New York, NY: Doubleday; 1994.
3. Coyle RG. *System Dynamics Modelling: A Practical Approach.* London, UK: Chapman & Hall; 1996.
4. Atun RA, Lebcir MR, McKee M, Habicht J, Coker RJ. Impact of joined-up HIV harm reduction and multidrug resistant tuberculosis control programmes in Estonia: system dynamics simulation model. *Health Policy.* 2007;81(2):207–217.
5. Lebcir RM, Atun RA, Coker RJ. System dynamic simulation of treatment policies to address colliding epidemics of tuberculosis, drug resistant tuberculosis and injecting drug users driven HIV in Russia. *J Oper Res Soc.* 2010;61:1238–1248.
6. Ahmad R, Zhu NJ, Lebcir RM, Atun R. How the health-seeking behaviour of pregnant women affect neonatal outcomes: findings of system dynamics modelling in Pakistan. *BMJ Glob Health.* 2019;4(2):e001242.
7. Darabi N, Hosseinichimeh N. System dynamics modeling in health and medicine: a systematic literature review. *Syst Dynam Rev.* 2020;36:29–73.
8. United Nations. UN Universal Declaration of Human Rights. https://www. un.org/en/universal-declaration-human-rights/
9. World Health Organization. Declaration of Alma-Ata. International Conference on Primary Health Care, Kazakhstan, USSR. Published 1978. http://www.who. int/publications/almaata_declaration_en.pdf
10. Hardin G. The tragedy of the commons. *Science.* 1968;162(3859):1243–1248.
11. Lloyd WF. *Two Lectures on the Checks to Population.* Oxford, UK: Oxford University; 1833.
12. The National Audit Office [UK]. Successful Commissioning Toolkit: Assessing Value for Money. https://www.nao.org.uk/successful-commissioning/general-principles/value-for-money/assessing-value-for-money/
13. Porter E, Teisberg EO. *Redefining Health Care: Creating Value-Based Competition on Results.* Boston, MA: Harvard Business School Press; 2006.

14. Schneider E, Sarnak DO, Squires D, Shah A, Doty MM. Mirror, mirror. *Commonwealth Fund*. Published July 14, 2017. https://www.commonwealthfund.org/publications/fund-reports/2017/jul/mirror-mirror-2017-international-comparison-reflects-flaws-and

15. Organisation for Economic Co-operation and Development. OECD Health Data 2020. https://www.oecd.org/health/health-data.htm

16. Kahneman D. *Thinking Fast and Slow*. New York, NY: Farrar, Straus and Giroux; 2011.

17. Argyris C, Schön D. *Organizational Learning II: Theory, Method and Practice*. Reading, MA: Addison Wesley; 1996.

18. Senge PM. *The Fifth Discipline: The Art and Practice of the Learning Organization*. New York, NY: Doubleday; 1990.

CHAPTER 8

1. Ferlie E, FitzGerald L, Wood M, Hawkins C. The (non) diffusion of innovations: the mediating role of professional groups. *Acad Manage J*. 2005;48:117–134.

2. Rogers EM. *Diffusion of Innovations*. New York, NY: Free Press; 2003.

3. Atun R, de Jongh T, Secci F, Ohiri K, Adeyi O. Integration of targeted health interventions into health systems: a conceptual framework for analysis. *Health Policy Plan*. 2010;25:104–111.

4. Foy R, MacLennan G, Grimshaw J, et al. Attributes of clinical recommendations that influence change in practice following audit and feedback. *J Clin Epidemiol*. 2002;55:717–722.

5. Fitzgerald L, Ferlie E, Hawkins C. Innovation in healthcare: how does credible evidence influence professionals? *Health Soc Care Community*. 2003;11(3):219–228.

6. Atun RA, Baeza J, Drobniewski F, Levicheva V, Coker R. Implementing WHO DOTS strategy in the Russian Federation: stakeholder attitudes. *Health Policy*. 2005;74(2):122–132.

7. Fitzgerald L, Ferlie E, Wood M, Hawkins C. Interlocking interactions: the diffusion of innovations in health care. *Human Relations*. 2002;55:1429–1449.

8. Locock L, Dopson S, Chambers D, Gabbay J. Understanding the role of opinion leaders in improving clinical effectiveness. *Social Sci Med*. 2001;53:745–757.

9. Plsek PE, Greenhalgh T. Complexity science: the challenge of complexity in health care. *BMJ*. 2001;323:625–628.

10. Coker RJ, Atun RA, McKee M. Health care system frailties and public health control of communicable disease on the European Union's new eastern border. *Lancet*. 2004;363:1389–1392.

11. Atun RA, Kyratsis I, Gurol I, Rados-Malicbegovic D, Jelic G. Diffusion of complex health innovations-implementation of primary care reforms in Bosnia and Herzegovina: a qualitative study. *Health Policy Plan*. 2007;22(1):28–39.

12. Denis JL, Hebert Y, Langley A, et al. Explaining diffusion patterns for complex health care innovations. *Health Care Manage Rev*. 2002;27:60–73.

13. Ferlie E, Fitzgerald L, Wood M. Getting evidence into clinical practice: an organisational behaviour perspective. *J Health Serv Res Policy*. 2000;5(2):96–102.

14. Kyratsis Y, Atun R, Phillips N, Tracey P, George G. Health systems in transition: identity work in the context of shifting institutional logics. *Acad Manage J*. 2017;60(2):610–641.

15. Atun RA, McKee M, Drobniewski F, Coker R. Analysis of how health system context influences HIV control: case studies from the Russian Federation. *Bull World Health Organ*. 2005;83(10):730–738.

16. Atun RA, Samyshkin YA, Drobniewski F, et al. Barriers to sustainable tuberculosis control in the Russian Federation. *Bull World Health Organ*. 2005;83(3):217–223.

17. Atun RA, Menabde N, Saluvere K, Jesse M, Habicht J. Implementing complex health innovations—primary health care reforms in Estonia: multimethod evaluation. *Health Policy*. 2006;79(1):79–91.

18. Coker RJ, Dimitrova B, Drobniewski F, et al. Tuberculosis control in Samara Oblast, Russia: institutional and regulatory environment. *Int J Tuberc Lung Disease*. 2003;7(10):920–932.

19. Pettigrew A, Ferlie E, McKee L. *Shaping Strategic Change: Making Change in Large Organizations: The Case of the National Health Service*. London, UK: SAGE; 1992.

20. West E, Barron DN, Dowsett J, Newton JN. Hierarchies and cliques in the social networks of health care professionals: implications for the design of dissemination strategies. *Soc Sci Med*. 1999;48:633–646.

21. Shortell SM, Bennett CL, Byck GR. Assessing the impact of continuous quality improvement on clinical practice: what will it take to accelerate progress? *Milbank Q*. 1998;76:593–624.

22. Barnsley J, Lemieux-Charles L, McKinney MM. Integrating learning into integrated delivery systems. *Health Care Manage Rev*. 1998;23:18–28.

23. Ferlie E, Gabbay J, Fitzgerald L, et al. Evidence-based medicine and organisational change: an overview of recent qualitative research. In: Ashburner L, ed. *Organisational Behaviour and Organisational Studies in Health Care: Reflections on the Future*. Basingstoke, UK: Palgrave; 2001.

24. Atun R. Health systems, systems thinking and innovation. *Health Policy Plan*. 2012;27:iv4–iv8.

25. Atun R, Menabde N. Health systems and systems thinking, In: Coker R, Atun R, McKee M, eds. *Health Systems and the Challenge Of Communicable Diseases: Experiences From Europe and Latin America*. London, UK: Open University Press; 2008.

26. Rogers EM. *Diffusion of Innovations*. 5th ed. New York, NY: Free Press; 2003.

27. Argyris C, Schön D. *Organizational Learning II: Theory, Method, and Practices*. New York, NY: Addison Wesley; 1996.

28. Meyer JW, Rowan B. Institutionalized organizations: formal structure as myth and ceremony. *Am J Sociol*. 1977;83:340–363.

29. Abrahamson EE. Managerial fads and fashions: the diffusion and refection of innovations. *Acad Manage Rev*. 1991;16(3):586–612.

30. Schumpeter JA. *The Theory of Economic Development: An Inquiry Into Profits, Capital, Credit, Interest, and the Business Cycle*. London, UK: Transaction; 1983.

31. Williamson O. *Corporate Control and Economic Behaviour*. New York, NY: Prentice-Hall; 1970.

32. Nelson RR, Peterhansl A., Sampat B. Why and how innovations get adopted: a tale of four models. *Ind Corp Change*. 2004;13(5):679–699.

33. Battista RN. Innovation and diffusion of health-related technologies: a conceptual framework. *Int J Technol Assess Health Care*. 1989;5(2):227–248.

34. Zucker LG. Institutional theories of organization. *Annu Rev Sociol*. 1987;13(1):443.

35. DiMaggio PJ. Interest and agency in institutional theory. In: *Institutional Patterns and Organizations: Culture and Environment*. Boston, MA: Pitman; 1987:3–22.
36. Greenaway J. How policy networks can damage democratic health: a case study in the government of governance. *Public Admin* 2007;85(3):717.
37. Dubé L, Addy NA, Blouin C, Drager N. From policy coherence to 21st century convergence: a whole-of-society paradigm of human and economic development. *Ann N Y Acad Sci*. 2014;1331:201–215.
38. Ostrum E. A general framework for analyzing sustainability of social-ecological systems. *Science*. 325:419–422.
39. Rogers EM. *Diffusion of Innovations*. 5th ed. New York, NY: Free Press; 2003.
40. Nohria N, Beer M. Cracking the code of change. Published May–June 2000. *Harvard Business Review*. https://hbr.org/2000/05/cracking-the-code-of-change
41. Ury W, Patton B. *Getting to Yes: Negotiating Agreement Without Giving In*. New York, NY: Penguin; 2011.
42. Daniels N, Sabin JE. *Setting Limits Fairly: Learning to Share Resources for Health*. New York, NY: Oxford University Press; 2008.

CHAPTER 9

1. Bradley EH, Taylor LA. *The American Health Care Paradox: Why Spending More Is Getting Us Less*. New York, NY: PublicAffairs; 2013.
2. Kuhn T. *The Structure of Scientific Revolutions*. Chicago, IL: University of Chicago Press; 1962.

INDEX

For the benefit of digital users, indexed terms that span two pages (e.g., 52–53) may, on occasion, appear on only one of those pages.

Tables, figures, and boxes are indicated by an italic *t*, *f* and *b* following the page number.

ethical evaluation methods, 46
Evans, R.G., 17
evidence-based practice, 60
experience, in value-for-money, 156–57, 157f, 158–60
external shocks. *See* context, health system

failure mode and effects analysis, 115b
fault tree analysis, 115b
feedback, misperception of, 9
fee-for-service systems, 40, 41t
financial protection, 51b
financing
    as health system function, 38–41, 40t, 41t
    health system described in terms of, 8, 18
    megatrends in all health systems, 59, 67
    system components most amenable to change, 117
first access care, 198
first impressions, establishing, 105–7, 106f
first-order change, 161–64, 163f, 172–73
fishbone diagram (cause-and-effect diagram), 112–13, 113f
Fisher, R., 185
5 Whys analysis, 110–12, 111f, 140
flow charts, 109, 129f, 129
focus groups, 116
force field analysis, 142, 187, 188f
forces driving change processes, 117–18
Forrester, Jay, 12, 59
framework for health system analysis. *See* health system analytic framework
functions, health system. *See also specific functions*
    and capacity, 180–81
    financing, 38–41, 40t, 41t
    governance and organization, 36–38, 37b
    measures of success related to, 132, 133t
    overview, 36
    resource management, 42–47, 44f, 47t
    system components most amenable to change, 116–18
    in systems view of health systems, 19–20

gaps
    associative processes to look for new ideas, 115–16
    closing in on, 95–96
    establishing first impressions and ideas, 106f, 106–7
    performance assessment, 85–89, 86f, 87t, 90f, 92
    prioritizing, 93–94, 94f
    understanding and describing problem and root causes, 107f, 107–15, 111f, 113f, 114f, 115b
Getting to Yes (Fisher, et al.), 185
goals, health system
    approaches to setting, 75–77, 76b
    country group meeting, 92–96, 94f
    deliverables, 96
    envisioning, 77–96
    exercises to help develop sense of, 80f, 80–83
    individual assignments, 91–92, 91t
    overview, 74–75, 83
    sizing up health system, 78–83
    spider diagrams, 85–89, 86f, 87t, 90f
    SWOT analysis, 83–84, 84t, 85t
    value-for-money and, 199
governance function, health system, 36–38, 37b, 117
group exercises. *See* small group exercises

happiness, as measure of quality of life, 63–64
Hardin, Garrett, 150–51
health
    for all as human right, 61–62
    determinants of, 2f, 2–4
    gains in health status of nations, 55–61
    good, in high-performing health systems, 6–7
    individual responsibility for, 2f, 4, 200, 215
    national priorities regarding, 87t
    relation to economic growth and development, 4–5, 5f
    in value proposition for health systems, 155–56, 156f, 160, 161f
health insurance. *See* insurance
health promotion services, 48

health protection services, 48
health system analytic framework
   conceptualizations of health
      systems, 17–19
   context, 22–36, 24*t*, 25*t*, 33*t*, 34*f*, 35*f*
   functions, 36–47, 37*b*, 40*t*, 41*t*,
      44*f*, 47*t*
   general discussion, 19–20
   individual assignment, 20–22, 21*t*
   objectives, 49*f*, 49–50, 51*t*
   outcomes, 51*b*, 51–52, 52*t*
   outputs, 47–49
   overview, 15–17, 16*f*
health system. *See also* megatrends in
      health systems; *specific aspects
      of health system design*; systems
      thinking
   attributes of successful, 195–201, 196*t*
   citizen responsibility, 214–15
   definitions and
      conceptualizations, 17–19
   evolution of, 53–55
   general discussion, 215–16
   health of population, 2*f*, 2–5, 5*f*
   high-performing, 6–7
   life stage development and
      opportunity for change,
      204*f*, 204–8
   overview, 1, 193
   reconceptualization, 208–14
   transformative change, 207–14
   truisms of design, 201–3
health technology assessment, 46, 47*t*
healthcare services. *See also* medical care;
      public health services; *specific
      related topics*
   improvements in delivery, 58–60
   relation to population health, 2*f*,
      2–4
   system components most amenable to
      change, 117
Healthy People 2030, 81, 82
high-performing health systems, 6–7.
      See also value-for-money
HIV pandemic, 171–72
hospitals
   effectiveness of, 58
   resistance to health system
      change, 195
human right, health for all as, 61–62

ideas, intervention
   associative processes to look for
      new, 115–16
   establishing first, 105–7, 106*f*
   narrowing down SIP, 99
   winnowing down, 119*f*, 119
impact score, SIP, 142
implementation. *See also* 7Cs model
   campaign plan, formulating,
      186–91, 188*f*
   general approach to testing for, 124–45,
      126*f*, 127*f*
   influences on, 168–69
   large group presentations, 191–92
   overview, 167–68
   planning, 187–91
   small group meeting, 191*b*, 191–92
   student work plan, 169
improvement planning. *See* D3A3
      model for improvement;
      intervention plans; systems
      improvement plan,
individual assignments. *See also*
      designing intervention
   applying D3A3 improvement model
      to SIP, 127–36, 128*t*, 129*f*, 131*f*,
      133*t*, 134*t*, 135*t*
   completing D3A3 model and choosing
      plan of action, 137–44, 138*b*,
      139*f*, 140*b*, 142*f*
   developing sense of system's vision
      and goals, 80*f*, 80–83
   drilling down on health system
      goals, 83–92, 84*t*, 85*t*, 86*f*, 87*t*,
      90*f*, 91*t*
   health system analysis, 15, 20–22, 21*t*,
      36, 42–43
   implementation, 169
   intervention plan, 101–4, 102*f*, 103*f*
   testing and refining SIP, 123
individual healthcare services. *See*
      medical care
individual responsibility for health, 2*f*, 4,
      200, 215
individualism
   and cohesiveness, 181*f*, 181
   in value proposition for health
      systems, 156–57, 157*f*, 158–60
inductive approach to creative
      thinking, 100

megatrends in all health systems
    effectiveness, 55–60, 60b
    efficiency, 65–71, 66b
    equity and accessibility to medical
        care, 61–65
    general discussion, 73
    overview, 53–55, 54f
    responsiveness and patient
        experience, 65
Mencken, H. L., 74
mental maps, 161
mental model of health system, 80f, 80
Michelangelo, 193
middle adopters, 178–79
mind mapping, 112, 113f, 116
ministries of health, role of, 37–38
misperception of feedback, 9
Model 1 thinking, 161–62, 163f
Model 2 thinking, 147, 161–66, 163f
model for improvement, 122.
        See also D3A3 model for
        improvement
modern medicine, 3
moral hazard, 68, 151–52

National Health Service (NHS), UK, 81,
        82, 159f, 202–3, 209–11
National Institute for Health and Care
        Excellence, UK, 60
national priorities, in performance
        assessment, 86f, 87t, 90f
national scorecard, 200–1
nations, gains in health status of, 55–61
need, defining, 203–4
Netherlands, 75–76, 159f, 160
normative considerations, resource
        management, 44–45

objectives, health system, 49f, 49–50,
        51t, 146–47. *See also* goals,
        health system
openness, to enhance
        cohesiveness, 185–86
opportunities
    for change, 204f, 204–8
    for health systems, 23, 35f, 35
    SWOT analysis, 83, 84, 85t, 92–93,
        106f, 106–7
opportunity costs, 142
Oregon Medicaid experiment, 211

organization function, health systems,
        36–38, 37b, 117
Organizational Learning II (Schön and
        Argyris), 185
organizational support to improve
        health status, 61–62
Ostrum, Elinor, 185
outcomes, health system
    assessing, 19–20, 51b, 51–52, 52t
    measures of success related to, 130,
        131f, 131–32, 133t, 134t
outputs, health system
    measures of success related to, 131f,
        131, 132, 133t
    overview, 47
    personal healthcare services, 48–49
    public health services, 48
    in systems view of health
        systems, 19–20

paradigmatic change, 163f,
        164–65, 208–14
Pareto charts, 114f, 114
patient experience, 65
patterns, looking for, 109
payment methods, provider, 39–40,
        41, 41t
PDSA workflow cycle, 126. *See also* D3A3
        model for improvement
performance
    rating with spider diagram, 85–92,
        86f, 87t, 90f, 93
    sources for assessing, 91t
personal experience, in value-for-
        money proposition, 156–57,
        157f, 158–60
personal healthcare services. *See*
        medical care
personal responsibility for health, 2f, 4,
        200, 215
PERT (program evaluation review
        technique) charts, 129f, 129
plans for change. *See* intervention plans
political environment, 24t, 25t, 27–28
population health
    defined, 51b
    determinants of, 2f, 2–4
    gains in, 55–61
    relation to economic growth and
        development, 4–5, 5f

Porter, Michael, 155
positioning map of stakeholders, 175, 177f
precision medicine, 48, 212
predictability, increasing, 124–25
predicting responses to changes, 135–36, 135t
prepared work force, importance of, 200
prevention, 48, 206
primary care, 58, 198
priority-setting. *See also* goals, health system
    accountability for reasonableness approach, 76b, 76
    and limits on healthcare spending, 70–71
    regarding gaps, 93–94, 94f
    and resource allocation, 42–47, 44f
    and value-for-money, 199, 202–4
private sources of funding, 39
private system, in UK, 209–10
private top–up option, 72, 200, 210
problems, understanding and describing, 107f, 107–15, 111f, 113f, 114f, 115b
program evaluation review technique (PERT) charts, 129f, 129
provider payment methods, 39–40, 41, 41t
public expectations, as threat to equity, 65
public health services
    as health system output, 48
    overview, 2–3
    precision, 48
    spider diagram performance assessment, 87t
    strengthening, 200
    trends in investment in, 69
public insurance schemes. *See* insurance
public sources of funding, 39
public–private mix, in UK NHS, 209–10
push models, 168

quality. *See* effectiveness
quality improvement (QI), 99
quality of life, 63–64

radar diagrams. *See* spider diagrams
rationing of medical care, 73.
    See also setting limits

Rawls, John, 71, 75
RCA (root cause analysis), 109–15, 111f, 113f, 114f, 115b, 139–40, 140b
readiness for change, 86f, 87t, 90f
reconceptualization, 164–65, 208–14
reductionist approach to systems, 9
reframing, 164
regulation
    cohesiveness through, 186
    in value-for-money proposition, 202
regulatory environment, 24t, 25t, 28
reimbursement megatrends, 59
resisters, 178–79
resource management
    developing sense of system's vision and goals, 81–82
    overview, 42–47, 44f, 47t
    system components most amenable to change, 117
    value-for-money and, 199
responsiveness, health system
    as essential parameter of success, 54f, 54–55
    overview, 49f, 50, 51t
    and patient experience, 65
    spider diagram performance assessment, 87t
right, health for all as, 61–62
risk
    attitudes toward taking, 178–79
    collective insurance as means to share, 62–63
    estimating, 143
Rogers, Everett, 167–68, 178–79
root cause analysis (RCA), 109–15, 111f, 113f, 114f, 115b, 139–40, 140b

Sabin, J.E., 185–86
salaries, as provider payment method, 39
satisfaction
    national priorities regarding, 87t
    user, as health system outcome, 51b
    in value proposition for health systems, 155–61, 156f, 157f, 158f, 159f, 161f, 207
saving lives, limits on, 212–13
Schön, D., 163, 164, 185
scientific discovery successes, 56–57
scorecard, national, 200–1

user satisfaction, 51*b*

value-for-money
    attributes of successful health
        systems, 195–201, 196*t*
    balancing act related to, 160–61, 161*f*
    challenges to, 194–95
    general discussion, 216
    life stage development and, 205–8
    national goals related to, 154–56, 156*f*
    new value proposition including
        satisfaction, 156–60, 157*f*,
        158*f*, 159*f*
    overview, 146–47
    truisms of health system design, 201–3
"veil of ignorance" concept, 71, 75

vision, health system, 81, 95–96. *See also*
    goals, health system
vision statement, formulating, 82–83

weaknesses, in SWOT analysis, 83, 84,
    84*t*, 92–93, 106*f*, 106–7
winnowing down ideas, 119*f*, 119
workforce, medical care, 59, 200
World Happiness Report, 63–64
World Health Organization (WHO), 8,
    17, 46, 61, 62

yield/effort tables, 119*f*, 119, 130,
    141, 142*f*

zone of opportunity, 204*f*, 207–8